MIRACLES IN MEDICINE

MIRACLES IN MEDICINE

M.W. MARTIN

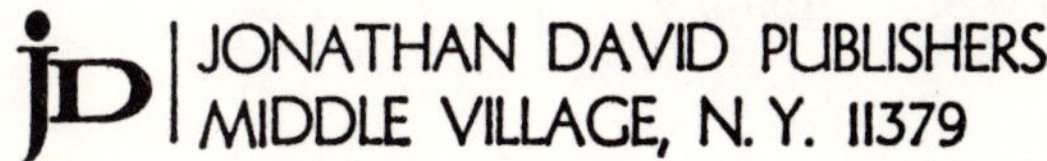

JONATHAN DAVID PUBLISHERS
MIDDLE VILLAGE, N.Y. 11379

MIRACLES IN MEDICINE
Copyright © 1974
by
M. W. Martin

No part of this book may be reproduced in any
manner without written permission from the
publishers.

Address all inquiries to:

JONATHAN DAVID PUBLISHERS
68-22 Eliot Avenue
Middle Village, New York 11379

Printed in the United States of America

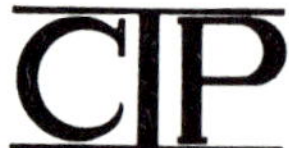

Library of Congress Cataloging in Publication Data

Martin, M W
   Miracles in medicine.

   1. Medicine—Addresses, essays, lectures.
2. Therapeutics—Addresses, essays, lectures.
I. Title. [DNLM: 1. Equipment and supplies—Popular
works. 2. Therapeutics—Popular works. 3. Transplantation—Popular works. WB300 M382m]
R117.M343   610   73-80419
ISBN 0-8246-0159-9

Table of Contents

ACKNOWLEDGMENTS

Many authorities were kind enough to take time from their busy professional schedules to contribute resource material for this volume, to submit excellent photographs, and to review the individual chapters pertinent to their specialties. My profound thanks are extended to the following medical men and scientists for their assistance, and particularly for their invaluable aid in reviewing the material.

Dr. Richard M. Ball, Plainfield, New Jersey.

Dr. Perry A. Berman, Bala Cynwyd, Pennsylvania.

Col. David G. Bowers, Lackland Air Force Base, Texas.

Dr. Carl T. Brighton, University of Pennsylvania School of Medicine, Philadelphia, Pennsylvania.

Dr. Harry J. Bunckc, Jr., University of California, San Francisco, California.

Dr. Michael Buonocore, Eastman Medical Center, Rochester, New York.

Dr. William B. Campbell, Ohio State University, Columbus, Ohio.

Dr. George E. Cartwright, College of Medicine, University of Utah, Salt Lake City, Utah.

Dr. J. Ryan Chandler, University of Miami School of Medicine, Miami, Florida.

Dr. Irving S. Cooper, St. Barnabas Hospital, Bronx, New York.

Dr. William E. Crisp, University of Arizona-Maricopa County General Hospital, Phoenix, Arizona.

Dr. Ross Davis, University of Miami School of Medicine, Miami, Florida.

Dr. Herbert Dedo, University of California, San Francisco, California.

Dr. A. F. Dwyer, Mater Misericordiae Hospital, Sydney, Australia.

Dr. William Feinbloom, New York, New York.

Dr. Gerhard H. Fromm, University of Pittsburgh School of Medicine, Pittsburgh, Pennsylvania.

Dr. Miles A. Galin, New York Medical College, New York, New York.

Dr. Gilbert H. Glaser, Yale University School of Medicine, New Haven, Connecticut.

Dr. William W.L. Glenn, Yale University School of Medicine, New Haven, Connecticut.

Dr. Leon Goldman, University of Cincinnati Medical School, Cincinnati, Ohio.

Dr. John E. Hall, Harvard Medical School, Boston, Massachusetts.

Dr. Kevin D. Harrington, University of California, San Francisco, California.

Dr. Basil S. Hilaris, Memorial Hospital for Cancer and Allied Diseases, New York, New York.

Mr. H.R. Hill, EMI Central Research Laboratories, London, England.

Dr. Alan F. Hofmann, Mayo Clinic, Rochester, Minnesota.

Dr. James F. Holland, Mount Sinai School of Medicine, New York, New York.

Dr. Charles A. Homsy, Methodist Hospital, Houston, Texas.

Dr. Julius H. Jacobson II, Mount Sinai Hospital, New York, New York.

Dr. Adrian Kantrowitz, Sinai Hospital, Detroit, Michigan.

Dr. Charles D. Kelman, Manhattan Eye, Ear and Throat Hospital, New York, New York.

Dr. John N. Kent, L.S.U. Medical Center, New Orleans, Louisiana.

Dr. Ian Knoetgen, University of Graz Neurosurgery Clinic, Graz, Austria.

Dr. Bertrand A. Kolles, St. Paul, Minnesota.

Dr. Norman Lasker, Jefferson Medical College, Philadelphia, Pennsylvania.

Dr. John K. Lattimer, College of Physicians and Surgeons, Columbia University, New York, New York.

Dr. Russell K. Lawson, University of Oregon Medical School, Portland, Oregon.

Prof. H.R. Lehneis, Institute of Rehabilitation Medicine, N.Y.U. Medical Center, New York, New York.

Dr. Martin I. Lewis, Queen of Angels Hospital, Los Angeles, California.

Dr. William A. Lieber, Lenox Hill Hospital, New York, New York.

Dr. Robert Machemer, Bascom Palmer Eye Institute, Miami, Florida.

Dr. Thomas Mallory, Columbus, Ohio.

Dr. John S. Najarian, Department of Surgery, University of Minnesota School of Medicine, Minneapolis, Minnesota.

Dr. Norman Orentreich, N.Y.U. School of Medicine, New York, New York.

Dr. James M. Ozenberger, Yale University School of Medicine, New Haven, Connecticut.

Dr. Anselmo Pineda, St. Mary's Hospital, Long Beach, California.

Dr. O.M. Reinmuth, University of Miami School of Medicine, Miami, Florida.

Dr. Hubert L. Rosomoff, University of Miami School of Medicine, Miami, Florida.

Dr. Joseph V.M. Ross, Berwick, Pennsylvania.

Dr. Antonio Scommegna, Michael Reese Hospital and Medical Center, Chicago, Illinois.

Dr. F. Brantley Scott, St. Luke's Episcopal Hospital, Houston, Texas.

Dr. H.H. Scudamore, Monroe Clinic, Monroe, Wisconsin.

Mr. Donald Selwyn, Director, National Institute for Rehabilitation Engineering, Pompton Lakes, New Jersey.

Dr. Arthur K. Shapiro, Payne Whitney Psychiatric Clinic, New York Hospital, New York, New York.

Prof. A.A. Sherwood, University of Sydney, Sydney, Australia.

Dr. Jerome A. Silbert, New York, New York.

Dr. Joseph V. Simone, St. Jude Children's Research Hospital, Memphis, Tennessee.

Dr. Albert Starr, University of Oregon Medical School, Portland, Oregon.

Dr. Alfred B. Swanson, Blodgett Memorial Hospital, Grand Rapids, Michigan.
Dr. Stanley Taub, New York Medical College, New York, New York.
Dr. Paul Tessier, Hospital Foch, Paris, France.
Dr. Noel R. Thompson, Middlesex Hospital, London, England.
Dr. Gordon Tinnis, William Beaumont Hospital, Royal Oaks, Michigan.
Dr. Robert Waters, Rancho Los Amigos Hospital, Downey, California.
Dr. Roger E. Wehrs, St. Francis Hospital, Tulsa, Oklahoma.
Dr. Fred W. Whitehouse, Henry Ford Hospital, Detroit, Michigan.
Dr. H.T.G. Williams, University of Alberta Hospital, Edmonton, Canada.
Dr. Gerald F. Winkler, Massachusetts General Hospital, Boston, Massachusetts.
Dr. Setrag A. Zacarian, Springfield Hospital Medical Center, Springfield, Massachusetts.

PHOTO CREDITS

American Medical Systems, Inc.; Dr. Frederick P. Dewer; National Institute for Rehabilitation Engineering; Martin's International Newsreel; Dr. Richard M. Ball; Dr. Kevin D. Harrington; Overly Manufacturing Co.; Telesensory Systems, Inc.; Dr. Roger E. Wehrs; Dr. Alan F. Hofmann; Dr. Carl T. Brighton; Mozes Engineering, Ltd.; Dr. Basil Hilaris; Dr. Setrag A. Zacarian; Dr. J.R. Chandler; EMI Central Research Laboratories; Dr. William B. Campbell; *Columbus Dispatch*; Dr. William A. Lieber; Australian Information Service; Dr. Robert Machemer; Prof. A.A. Sherwood; Bascom Palmer Eye Institute; Cardiodynamics, Inc.; BIPS; Hugh Steeper (Roehampton) Ltd.; Dr. John N. Kent; IDANT Corp.; Visualtek; Electro Labs; Medtronics; Prof. H.R. Lehneis, N.Y.U. Medical Center; Dr. Ross Davis; Stimtech Corp.; Cavitron Surgical Systems; National Research Council of Canada; Helper Industries, Inc.; Dynatch Cryomedical Co.; Ohio Medical Products; American Cancer Society; Dr. Thomas H. Mallory; Zimmer, U.S.A.; Dr. Stanley Taub; Dr. Leon Goldman; Dr. Norman Orentreich; Dr. Gerald F. Winkler; American Optometric Assoc.; Dr. Stuart C. Grant; Dr. Ian Knoetgen; American Medical Products Corp.; Dr. John K. Lattimer (*Urologic Procedures* 2:1); Dr. Julius H. Jacobson II; Dr. William Feinbloom; Alza Corp.; Dr. Antonia Scommegna; Life Support, Inc.; Dr. Noel Thompson; Dr. Paul Tessier; Dr. Harry J. Buncke, Jr.; Dr. J. Ryan Chandler; Hadassah; Dr. James M. Ozenberger; Bionic Instruments, Inc.; Dr. Perry A. Berman; Dr. Fred W. Whitehouse; Dr. Michael Buonocore; Dr. Irving S. Cooper; Dr. Miles A. Gallin, New York Medical College; Institute of Rehabilitation Medicine, N.Y.U. Medical Center; Dr. Alfred B. Swanson; Col. David G. Bowers; University of Utah; Overly Manufacturing Co.; Dr. Albert Starr; Dr. Anselmo Pineda; Sybron Corp.; Dr. Adrian Kantrowitz; Dr. Russell K. Lawson; Price Bros. & Co. Ltd.; Dr. William H. Harris; Tri-Tronics Laboratory, Inc.; Dr. Gerhard H. Fromm; A.G. Siemens; Rancho Los Amigos Hospital; Roche *Image*; Japan Information Service.

MIRACLES IN MEDICINE

FOREWORD

The purpose of *Miracles in Medicine* is to inform the average reader of some of the many "miracles" in medicine that have occurred in recent years. The volume describes methods of treatment as well as actual cures and discoveries that have helped, or are helping, many people. We call them miracles because for so many sick and suffering individuals almost all hope had vanished—and has now been renewed.

The purpose of the book is *not* to serve as a textbook on medicine; nor is the patient to use it as a guide to treat himself. It does not discuss the causes of a disease. It assumes that those most directly affected, or deeply interested, will consult their own physician, or will turn to some of the more technical books now available on many of the subjects under discussion. They may also write directly to the parties who have developed or invented the new processes, cures or medications. These names and addresses have been given wherever available.

M. W. MARTIN

1. NEW IMPLANT PERFORMS FUNCTIONS OF THE BLADDER

ABOUT ONE AND ONE-HALF million Americans suffer from abnormal or totally ineffective bladders. Some have no control over the bladder function at all, while others pass urine through various implanted medical devices, or surgically-prepared openings in the body. In the latter cases, there is the ever-present danger of infection and kidney damage and, quite often, repeated operations are needed to keep the bladder working or the patient will die.

Now, two physicians and an engineer have come up with an artificial sphincter (the muscle which operates the bladder), which, according to one of them, "can perhaps benefit 80% of the 1.5 million sufferers." The two doctors are Dr. F. Brantley Scott, Chief of Urology at St. Luke's Episcopal Hospital in Houston, Texas, and Dr. William Bradley, Professor of Neurology at the University of Minnesota. The engineer is Dr. Gerald Timm.

The artificial sphincter is implanted in the neck of the bladder. It consists of a reservoir pouch made of plasticized dacron mesh, plastic tubing, a plasticized rubber cuff with a check valve, and squeeze bulbs.

The cuff is implanted around the urethra (the canal which leads from the bladder to discharge the urine) and is connected to the squeeze bulbs with plastic tubing. Up and in

3

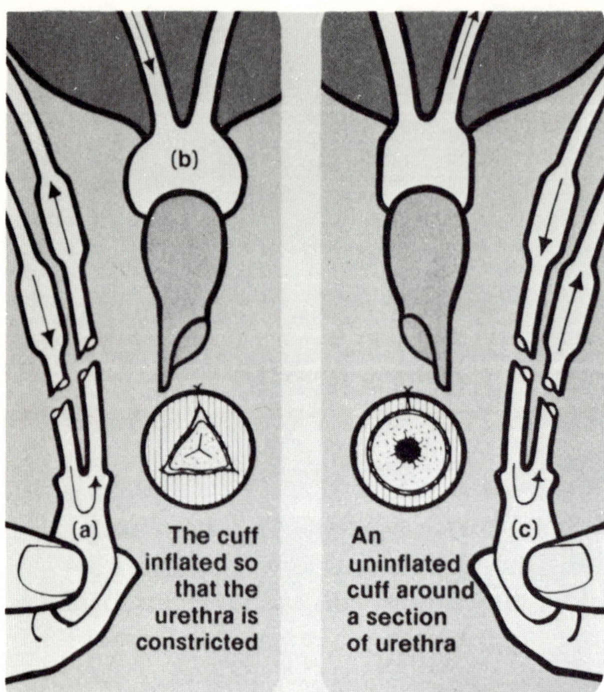

The artificial sphincter syste (left) can be implanted in bot male and female patients ar stimulates the urinary sphin ter to constrict the ureth without contacting the urina stream. The compressive for of the cuff is regulated by tl fluid storage and transfer sy tem shown.

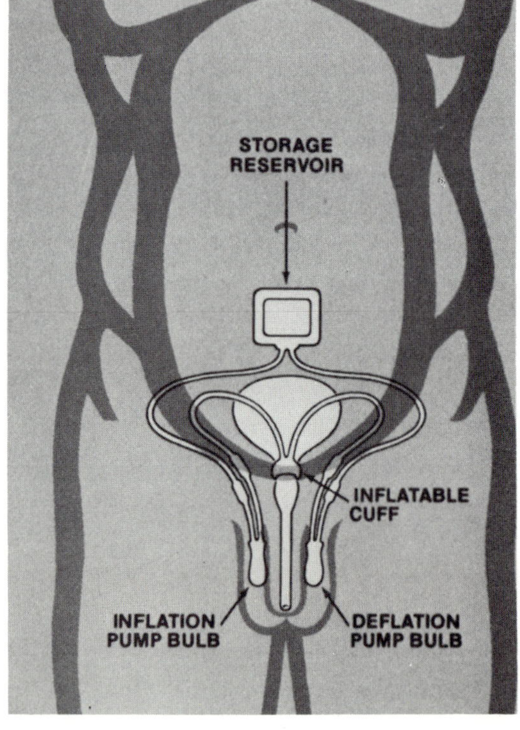

back of the cuff is placed the reservoir which is connected to the squeeze bulbs with another set of plastic piping (see drawing on oppposite page). The squeeze bulbs act as pumps, inflating or deflating the cuff, and causing the urine to discharge from the bladder. The reservoir is filled with radiopaque fluid (which can be seen with X-rays) which circulates down to the pumping cuff and back again, allowing the artificial sphincter to be easily monitored with X-rays to make sure that it is working properly.

The squeeze bulbs, which act as pumps, are placed in the scrotum (or the labia, in a woman) where they can be easily operated by the patient with his fingers. The bulbs are moveable and do not interfere with sex or sports. The patient starts or stops voiding by squeezing the opposite bulbs.

This new implant can, of course, serve only the patient who still has sensation left, and can feel when he has to pass urine. Those who have no feeling can also use it, but must void according to a time schedule.

The Scott-Bradley team is now testing an artificial sphincter with an electrostimulation device that controls the flow of urine on a time basis by fingertip pressure, and they are also working on a unit which will be equipped with a sensor which will be triggered by the built-up volume of urine in the bladder. With the bladder full and ready to be voided, the sensor will send out a beep signal alerting the wearer to urinate.

When fully developed and operating, these devices will bring immense relief to persons whose continence mechanism is damaged, such as prostatectomy patients, accident victims, and those with neurologic diseases—paraplegics, multiple sclerosis victims, Parkinsonism and spina bifida patients.

2. CAN OXYGEN FIGHT SENILITY?

THE USE OF HYPERBARIC OXYGEN in medical treatment is over thirty years old. It was first used to treat decompression sickness (bends) suffered by deep-water divers. The treatment consists of placing the patient in a special, air-tight chamber called a *hyperbaric chamber* (decompression chamber) and making him breathe (through a mask) pure oxygen, while, at the same time, the air pressure in the chamber is increased to several times normal air pressure.

Breathing in pure oxygen while being subjected to increased air pressure increases the supply of oxygen in the blood. Medically, the treatment is called *hyperbaric oxygenation*. Hyperbaric oxygenation has proved very effective in the treatment of carbon monoxide poisoning, gas gangrene, bed sores (cutaneous ulcers), air embolism, and smoke inhalation —to mention just some of the maladies which yield to the increased supply of oxygen in the blood produced by the treatment. Other conditions for which the treatment has been used are arthritis, burns, strokes and senility.

The use of hyperbaric oxygenation in the treatment of senility was first reported in 1969, by Dr. Eleanor Jacobs, of the State University of New York. Her report of "dramatic" improvement in 13 senile patients given oxygen under high

---

Additional material touching on this subject can be found in chapter 59.

pressure (OHP) opened the door for reports from other investigators who have been working on this treatment.

One of the strongest advocates of the use of OHP in treating the senile is Dr. Edgar End, of the Medical College of Wisconsin in Milwaukee. Dr. End has also been the director, since 1940, of the Milwaukee County Hyperbaric Unit, the oldest decompression chamber in continuous use in the nation. (A world-wide directory of hyperbaric chambers can be obtained from the U.S. Navy Supervisor of Diving, Department of the Navy, Washington, D.C. 20390.)

Dr. End has been treating senility with OHP since 1965, and he is very enthusiastic about its effectiveness. He has treated nearly 100 aged patients with OHP and he finds the treatment safe, effective, painless and rewarding. "In addition to the improvement in mental function experienced in the majority of the patients I have treated," says Dr. End, "there has been improvement in their feeling of well-being. They have eaten, slept, and socialized better. Their dispositions have improved and their interests have broadened and become more rewarding." Dr. End believes that OHP is a most promising method of fighting senility.

Dr. End's treatment for senility varies depending on the condition of the individual being treated, but in general, it consists of 10 to 30 daily, half-hour sessions in the chamber. The air pressure inside the chamber is maintained at about two-and-a-half times normal air pressure, and the pure oxygen—the "medicine"—is breathed in by mask.

Another area of hyperbaric oxygenation about which Dr. End is very enthusiastic is in the treatment of strokes. He finds OHP superbly effective in reducing the severity and duration of symptoms.

Since a hyperbaric chamber is an extremely costly installation (very close to a million dollars), and is very expensive to operate (about $250,000 a year), their number is not very large. Those in operation are insufficient to take care of even a fraction of the nation's aged and senile; nor can they take care of even a small fraction of the yearly toll of 60,000 stroke victims. But there are probably a sufficient number of installations around the nation to make it possible for readers who might want to try this "wonder drug." Of course, the treatment has to be prescribed by a physician.

3. OPERATION TO CORRECT BUNIONS

A SIMPLE, EASY operation to correct bunions has been devised by two Canadian surgeons from the Toronto General Hospital: Drs. Frederick P. Dewer and James D. Rathbun.

The procedure, called an *oblique transposition osteotomy*, is performed on the bone of the big toe.

Bunions are relatively common to women and they are usually traceable to a big toe deformity which starts in adolescence. Its technical description is *hallux valgus*. Hallux valgus is a deviation of the big toe toward the outer side of the foot. It causes the big toe to "hook over" its neighbor slightly, while the outer side of the foot, immediately at the end of the big toe, curves outwards. Pressure caused by hallux vulgus causes a bunion.

In the operation to correct the bunion, the bone is shortened, the foot narrowed, and the big toe is brought into alignment with its neighbor. Once the hallux valgus is corrected, the pressure is relieved and the bunion recedes by itself.

The Canadian team has performed about 40 of these operations in the last 14 years on patients aged 11 to 34. But Dr. Rathbun says, it is best to operate in early adolescence, because by the time a person reaches 20 he usually has a considerably atrophied first joint in the big toe, and even though

---

Additional material touching on this subject can be found in chapter 62.

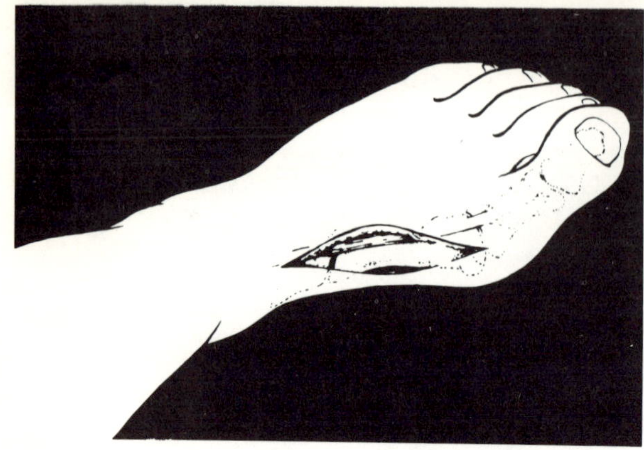

Correcting bunions with an oblique transposition osteotomy. The first step (left) exposes the first metatarsal.

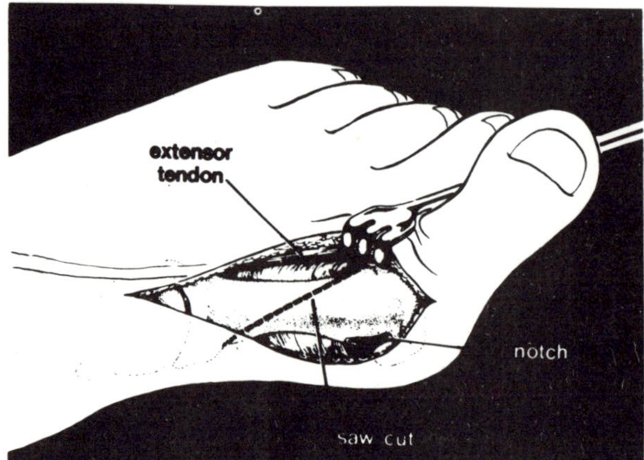

Pulling the extensor tendon of the big toe out of the way.

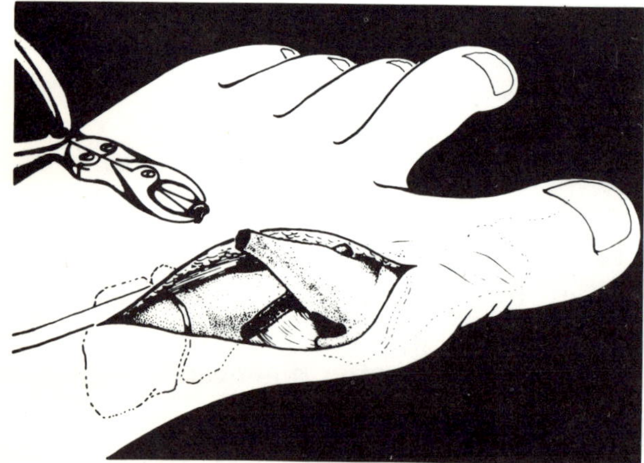

Transposition of the bones.

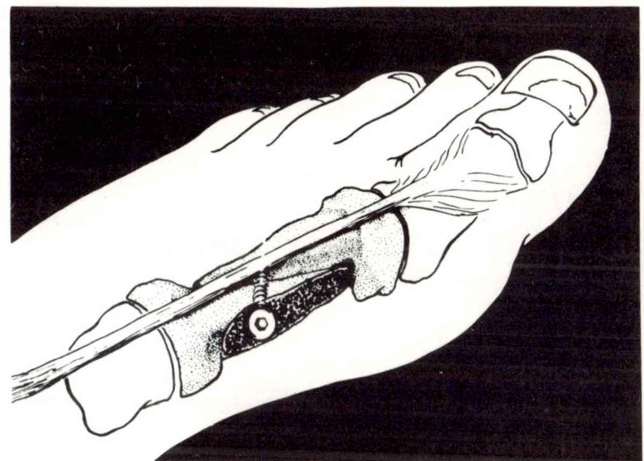

Fixation of the transposed bones with a screw.

the operation corrects the hallux vulgus, the joint later becomes stiff.

In the actual procedure, a cut is made on the side of the foot, exposing the bone leading to the big toe. A notch is cut into the bone and then the bone is cut through diagonally, at exactly the right angle to the sole of the foot. The cut ends of the bone are then lifted up, and shortened by trimming about ⅛″ to ¼″ off the tips.

Once shortened, the bony pieces are transposed one over the other, and fastened to each other with one or two screws. The transposed end of the piece which was previously in the back now fits into the notch which was cut into the front of the bone. The bones have to be shortened enough to allow the tendon controlling the big toe to lie straight along the newly formed straight bone without subjecting it to too much tension.

After surgery the patients are placed in a snug non-weight-bearing leg cast for about six weeks after which they can wear wooden sandals. It takes about three to four months for the transposed bones to grow back together.

4. A MEDICAL AID
FOR THE TRAVELER ABROAD

IF YOU'RE TRAVELING abroad, an excellent medical helper is available that can help you, should you need medical attention in a foreign country, whose language you can't speak.

The helper is a unique, extremely practical medical guidebook, called the *Pictorial Interpreter of Medicine.* It contains more than 200 multi-colored illustrations which completely replace the spoken word in most routine medical consultations.

The guidebook was written by Dr. Jack Adams-Ray, a Swedish professor of surgery who was forced, due to an accident, to endure a long recuperative hospital stay in a foreign country (Russia) where he experienced the usual despair caused by his inability to communicate even elementary needs to doctors and nurses. This additional burden on him and other alien patients made him decide to do something about it.

It took Dr. Adams-Ray a year of work with the help of an expert illustrator to produce the *Interpreter.* The idea was to provide doctors, nurses and hospital staff a means whereby a foreign patient's condition could be expressed without resorting to actual spoken words. This method relied completely on the universal language of pictures. The guidebook solved the problem.

PATIENTEN ÖNSKAR
THE PATIENT WISHES
LE MALADE DEMANDE
DER PATIENT WÜNSCHT
EL PACIENTE DESEA

IL PAZIENTE DESIDERA
PACIJENT ŽELI
Ο ΑΡΡΟΣΤΟΣ ΖΗΤΑ
POTILAS HALUAA

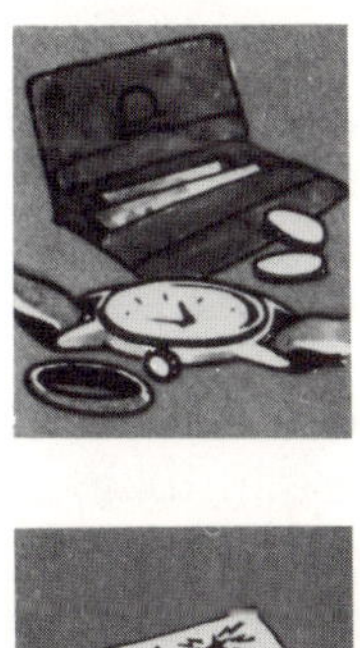
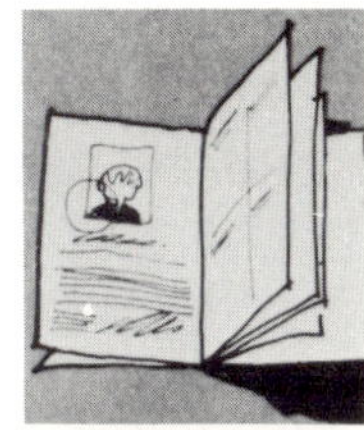
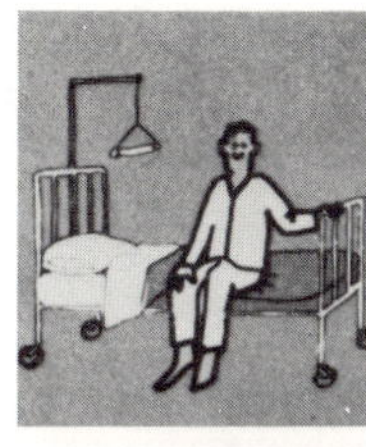
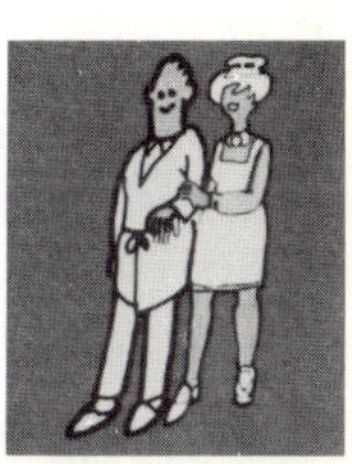
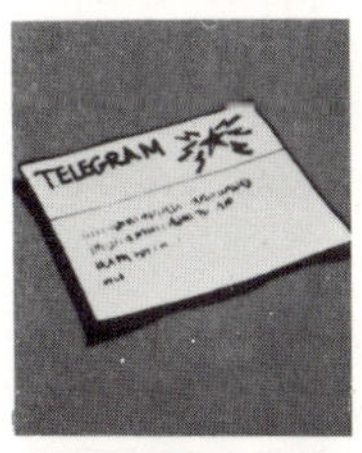

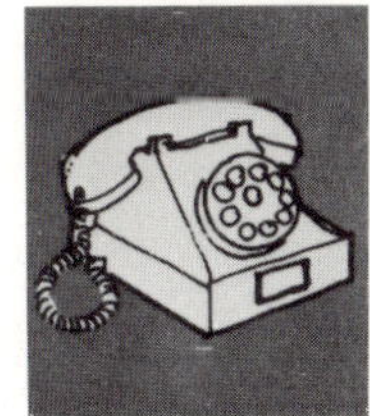

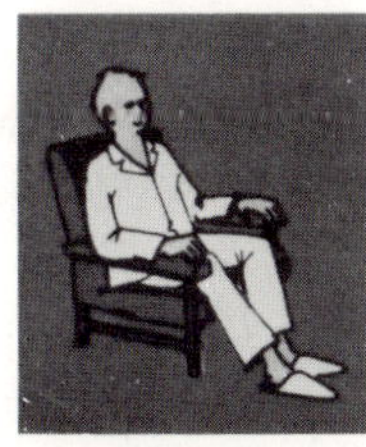
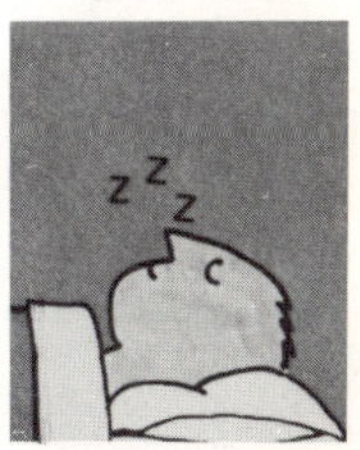
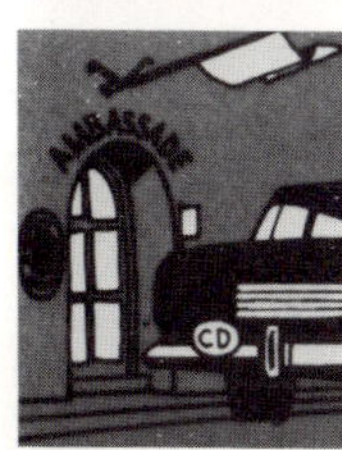

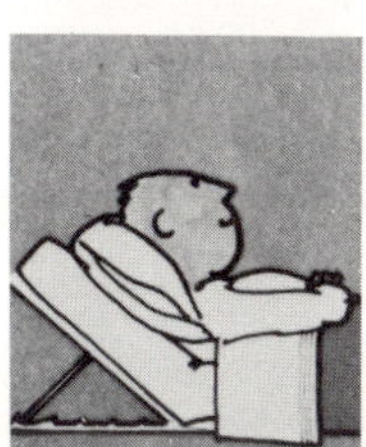
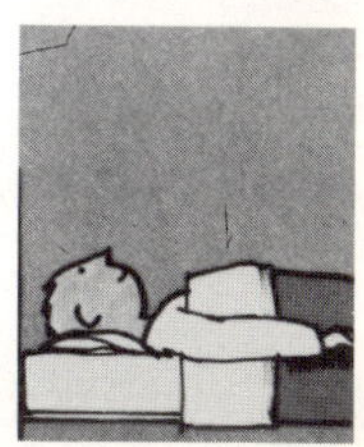

14   15

A few sample pages from the *Interpreter*, taken from the section, "The Patient Wishes." To indicate his wishes, the patient points to the appropriate box.

The *Interpreter* now contains a total of eight words in four color-coded indexed sections entitled: The patient wishes: The nurse says; The doctor asks; The patient says. These headings are translated into ten languages.

From now on, whenever a patient (anywhere in the world)

consulting a doctor has language difficulties, his ailment can be located without uttering a word. Even afflictions such as pain are easily described and detailed through the *Interpreter* thanks to its vivid full color and expressive anatomical and symbolic drawings. Likewise, a patient can express his needs and wants quickly and simply without any anxiety and stress.

Even in this country, the guidebook is ideal for people unable to speak during post operative conditions. Without doubt, the deaf and the orally handicapped especially will find it useful.

The slim, 44-page, soft-cover booklet, is only about four by eight inches and easily slips into a coat pocket or a handbag. It costs $1.75 and can be obtained from T.M. Visual Industries, Inc., 25 West 45 Street, New York, New York 10036.

5. A SPACE-AGE VOICE FOR SPASTICS

OUR SPACE PROGRAM TECHNOLOGY has given a severely spastic 10-year-old boy in New York the power of understandable speech.

The boy has an *athetoid* form of cerebral palsy; he has no voluntary control over his legs, arms or hands, and has lived his life in a wheelchair. Until now, his speech has been almost incomprehensible. He has difficulty coordinating his breathing with his speech, and in controlling the movements of his tongue and lips.

Now, he has been helped with a speech clarifier that takes much of the effort out of his talking—he does not need to take so many deep breaths, nor try to speak louder. This makes his speech more coherent and allows him to concentrate on correcting his pronunciation, and that, in turn, makes his speech even clearer.

The clarifier is a practical, cheap electronic speech aid that filters the voice, clarifies it, and amplifies it. It was developed by the National Institute for Rehabilitation Engineering in Pompton Lakes, N.J. by telephone engineers at the American Telephone and Telegraph Company from data derived for processing communications from spacecraft.

Telephone engineers were trying to find the most efficient

Additional material touching on this subject can be found in chapters 41, 78 and 83

way to transmit and recreate intelligible speech from spacecraft to earth, and in the course of this work they developed ways to eliminate distortion and background noise. Their results were taken up by engineers at the National Institute for Rehabilitation Engineering at Pompton Lakes, New Jersey. These engineers designed the miniaturized device which filters out unwanted voice frequencies, and boosts others to help the impaired speech of each of the handicapped individuals tested.

The device is simple and unobtrusive. It consists of a small microphone, attached to a head-band or eyeglass temple bar, and a battery-powered processing unit, contained in a tiny box fastened to a wheelchair, or worn in the user's clothing. The clarifier is intended to help people with speech disabilities that cannot be corrected medically or by speech therapy. Others who might be able to use it include persons with Parkinsonism, multiple sclerosis, amytrophic lateral sclerosis, and even those with certain types of injury to the vocal cords or vocal cord paralysis. It does not create speech for *total* laryngectomees, but does amplify and clarify speech for *partial* laryngectomees—or for totals using esophageal speech.

A measure of usefulness of the new device can be gathered from the experience of the first user. Originally, the boy was committed to a mental institution because doctors thought his inability to speak intelligibly was the result of mental retardation. In fact he has an above average IQ; he now goes to the hospital school and has learned to use a typewriter, operating the keys with a stick attached to a headband. His speech is still sometimes difficult to follow, but the clarifier has made it possible for him to hold conversations and take part in activities in school or at the hospital. He even sang a solo in the hospital's Christmas concert. Since Eddie Bartz received his speech aid, hundreds more have been successfully fitted to

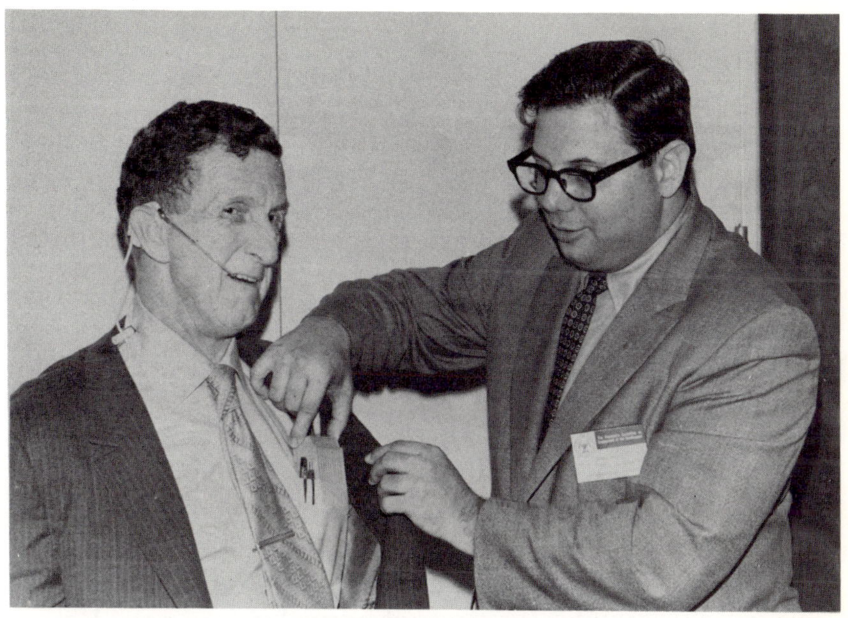

The new speech aid being demonstrated.

people all over the U.S. Experience to date, NIRE reports, is success with 35% to 40% of cerebral palsied, 60% of ALS and MS patients, and 85% to 90% of those with Parkinson s disease.

Inquiries may be addressed to: The National Institute for Rehabilitation Engineering, Pompton Lakes, N.J. 07442.

6. CEMENTING CANCER-CAUSED FRACTURES

NOT ALL BONE FRACTURES are caused by accidents. A kind of bone fracture called a *pathologic fracture* occurs in persons suffering from severe bone cancer. The cancer destroys the bone by "eating" it away. So much substance of the bone is lost to cancer that the bone becomes very weak and can break under the stress of normal movements. For example, a person suffering from this advanced stage of bone cancer in the humerus (upper arm bone) can break the arm just turning over in bed.

Persons with advanced bone cancer have a short life expectancy. Only 30% survive for one year or longer. The problem with these patients is to make their remaining life time bearable—relieving the pain caused by the broken bone and allowing them to regain its use, if possible. Conventional repair of broken bones is difficult, if possible at all. The bones are often so extensively replaced by tumor that they can no longer heal. Often, the only remedy is immobilization in a plaster cast or confinement in traction either of which often leads to a painful, accelerated downhill course for the patient.

Now, teams of doctors in several institutions have reported using *methylmethacrylate,* a cement used in hip surgery, to

---

Additional material touching on this subject can be found in chapters 12, 18, 26 and 40.

stabilize these cancer-caused fractures. They find that this rapidly setting cement fills space in diseased bones, locks the conventional fixation devices in place, and allows cancer patients to use their arms or walk again without pain.

This cement is not a glue—it does not glue the broken bones together, but it acts as a substitute for the destroyed bone, serving as "stock" for insertion of the screws and nails that unite the broken bones. (Chemically, the cement is the same substance which is known to the general public as Plexiglas and Lucite.)

The use of this cement has been reported from the Columbia-Presbyterian Medical Center in New York; the Mayo Clinic in Rochester, Minnesota; and the University of California School of Medicine in San Francisco. Dr. Richard M. Ball of the Columbia-Presbyterian team, and now at Rutgers Medical School, reported that of the 15 cases treated, all patients were relieved of pain, but that the restoration of the use of the limbs was uneven. Some patients did not improve at all; others regained use of their arms or were able to walk painlessly.

On the West Coast, Dr. Kevin D. Harrington, of the University of California team, reported a striking improvement in the 30 treated patients, 28 of them regaining their ability to walk in an average of seven days.

Despite the good experience and the lack of any side-effects or complications, all the doctors involved stress that many questions remain unanswered, including that of how long the cemented bones may be expected to survive the stress of weight-bearing. Another question is whether any healing occurs. According to the Columbia team, there is no evidence of healing; possibly, they report, the cement prevents healing. However, according to California's Dr. Harrington, these questions are not important, because of the nature of the disease being treated: advanced cancer in persons of short life expectancy. The aim of the the treatment, says Dr. Harrington, is the "immediate restoration of a painless and well-functioning limb."

7. HEART PACEMAKER
RECHARGES WITHOUT SURGERY

HIS HOBBY of making remote-control gliders helped Dr. Hans-Juergen Wanjura, a young German physician at West Berlin's University Clinic, invent a heart pacemaker which can be recharged while still in the patient's body, without the need of an operation.

The new pacemaker is about the size of a box of wooden matches, and weighs only slightly over two ounces. It is different from other types of pacemakers in that it can remain in the body of the patient for an indefinite time.

The Wanjura pacemaker is implanted in the abdominal wall and is connected to the heart. It is powered by fully charged nickel-cadmium batteries which release their power gradually. When the batteries are exhausted, they are recharged by simply holding the charger—a small, high-frequency generator—against the body, over the implanted pacemaker. The German battery manufacturer claims that, if properly handled, they can be recharged as many as 300 times.

Since present-day pacemaker batteries must be replaced by surgery about every 18 months, scientists have toyed with the idea of a pacemaker which can be recharged through the skin

Additional material touching on this subject can be found in chapters 24, 32, 46, 84, 94, 96, 98 and 99.

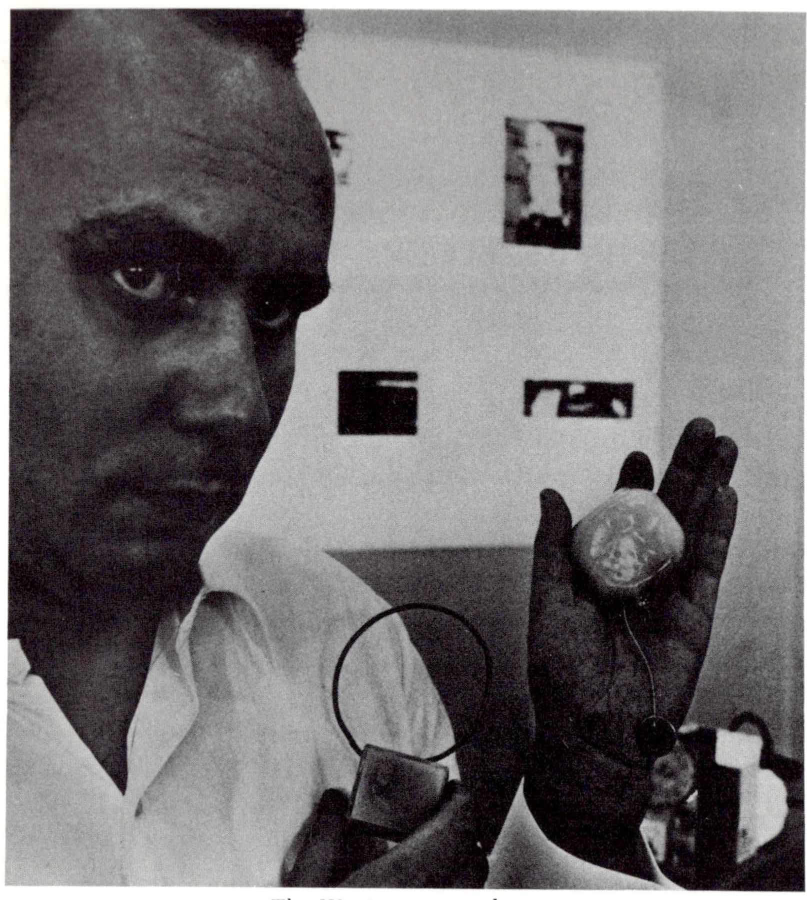

The Wanjura pacemaker.

with radio waves. But, until now, no practical device was ever built. It still remains to be seen whether the Wanjura pacemaker will turn out to be fully reliable.

A pacemaker similar to that of Dr. Wanjura was developed by a Columbia University engineer and a team of doctors from the Weizmann Institute of Science in Israel. This three-ounce unit is also powered by nickel-cadmium batteries, which can be recharged by radio waves picked up by a built-in receiving cell. It announces a dying battery by resonating (which is detected by radio waves) or by speeding up the pulse. It also has a built-in safety device to prevent an explosion in cases where the batteries had been accidentally overcharged.

The three-ounce unit can be recharged at night, while the patient is asleep. It can be done either at home or in the hospital. The recharging session takes from eight to ten hours.

This new pacemaker has been tested on animals, and although the experiments have been successful, the unit has not yet been implanted in humans. Additional animal tests are still being carried out. The pacemaker will be made in this country by Electro-Catheter Corp., Rahway, New Jersey.

8. A STAND-UP WHEEL CHAIR

AN IMAGINATIVE, NEW wheel chair which permits most users to stand or sit without someone's assistance is now available throughout the United States and Canada. The new chair helps users stand whenever they wish by using their own natural body motions.

To stand up, the user simply swings the foot rests down to the floor, then releases a set of knobs protruding from the seat rails, and he leans forward. This action frees automatic locks and permits concealed spring pistons, adjusted to the user's weight, to lift the individual gently into any desired position up to 10 degrees from vertical. Safety belts at the knees and across the hips provide insurance against mishaps without seriously restricting natural movements.

To reverse the procedure, the user simply unlocks the release knobs and leans backward.

The new chair was originally designed for paraplegics, but it is also useful for those with severe pulmonary disease (who cannot stand the strain of rising and sitting), arthritics, cardiac invalids, amputees, and those with neuromuscular disorders.

Psychologically, the benefits of the chair, which comes in many color combinations, including bright blue and yellow, are very important. Such functions as using the toilet or using

---

Additional material touching on this subject can be found in chapters 37 and 66.

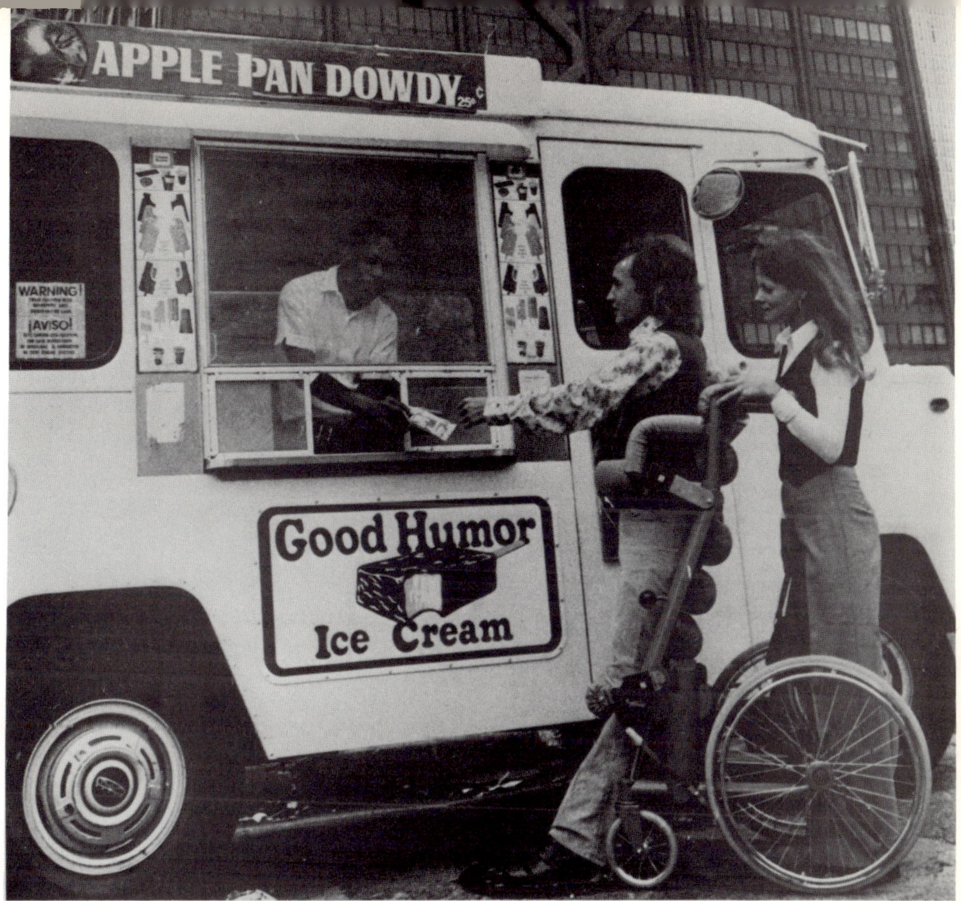

a pay phone, suddenly become normal routine once again. Users are able to "face the world" again at eye-level; and can perform many functions that are best performed in a standing position. Because of this new invention some invalids are now able to return to former occupations.

The chair is only 28 inches wide, which means that it can go through standard door openings. It weighs about 55 pounds, allowing it to be moved easily in and out of a car. Instead of folding, it splits into two sections that fit the back seat of any car—even a Volkswagen.

The chair is made by the Overly Manufacturing Co., of Greensburgh, Pennsylvania, and is sold through surgical supply houses at $550.

Readers are cautioned not to purchase this chair without prior approval by their physician, because some persons raising from a sitting to a standing position sometimes suffer a blackout.

9. CAMERA HELPS BLIND TO "READ" PRINTING

A "READING" MACHINE for the blind, invented several years ago by Dr. James Bliss of California, is now being produced in quantity and is available for purchase from Telesensory Systems, Inc., of Palo Alto, California. The device is called the *Optacon.* With the Optacon machine, a blind person can read ordinary, printed letters—just as you are now reading this page.

The Optacon machine has two units. One unit is called the *reader* and the other is called the *feeler.* The reader is a small camera, about the size of a pocket knife, attached to the feeler with a cord. This camera, which works very much like a tiny TV camera, photographs each printed letter and sends the pictures to the feeler. The camera photographs one printed letter at a time.

The feeler is a small box which contains the electronic equipment that runs the machine. The box has an opening into which the blind person can insert his fingertips. Inside that opening is a small pad, just the size of one fingertip. This pad has 144 tiny metal rods in it, and each rod can vibrate by itself. The movement of the rods can be felt by the blind person with the fingertip.

The photograph of the printed letter (taken by the reader camera) is converted electronically into a drawing of that letter and the tiny rods automatically form the shape of that

---

Additional material touching on this subject can be found in chapters 21, 25, 30, 36, 56 and 70.

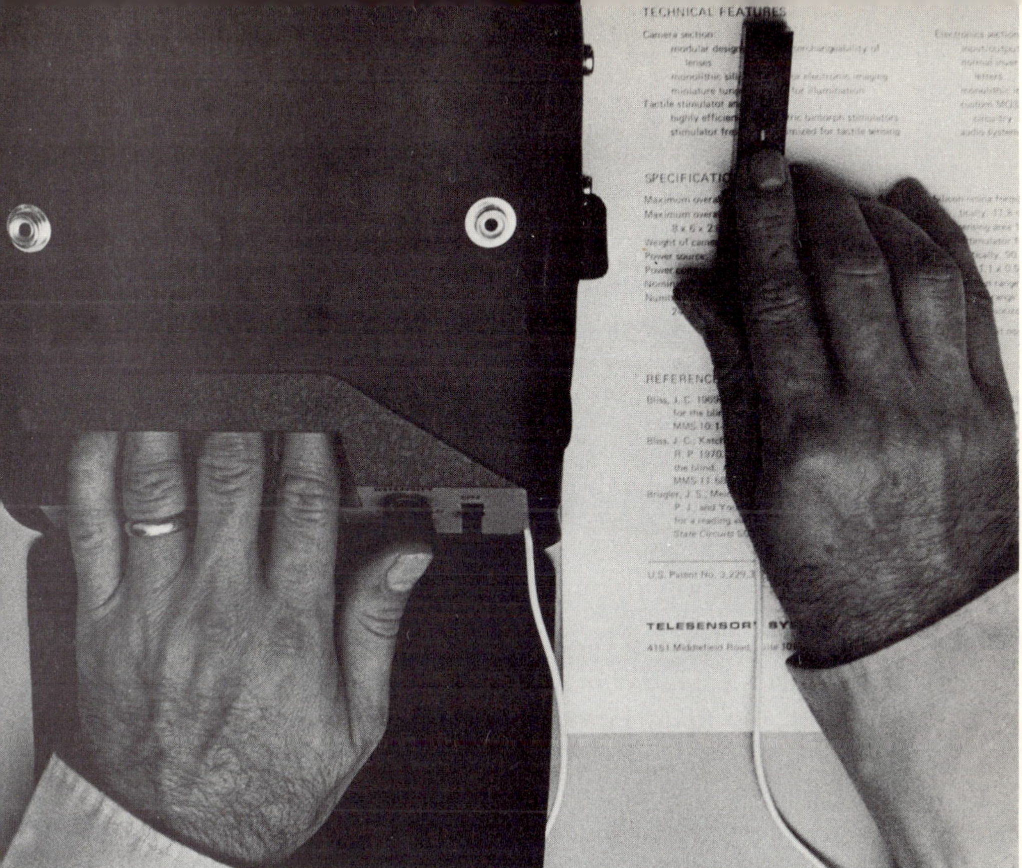

The Optacon reader. The person using the machine rests his thumb on the stimulator intensity control knob while his index finger is on the stimulator.

letter by vibrating. The blind person using the feeler can feel the outline of the letter vibrate on his fingertip. An "a" *feels* to him what an "a" *looks* like to you.

It takes time to learn to use the machine, but after a few weeks the blind person can recognize each letter photographed by the reader. A blind person experienced in using the Optacon can read 50 to 80 words per minute. The great advantage of the Optacon is that it eliminates the need of converting printing to braille, and makes the blind person more competitive in a sighted world.

About 200 Optacon units have been built and work is now under way to produce an even more compact and simple model. The Optacon presently sells for just under $4,000 and the price includes an intensive training class which the company operates in Palo Alto. Various training aids are also available.

10. EARDRUM TRANSPLANTS

THE EARDRUM is very small, but very important. It is slightly over a quarter of an inch across and is shaped like a cone with the point facing into the head.

The eardrum is so extremely important because if it is defective, we cannot hear. When sound waves touch it, it vibrates and carries the sound to other parts of the ear.

The newest round of transplantation is the replacement of diseased parts of the ear, in order to restore hearing.

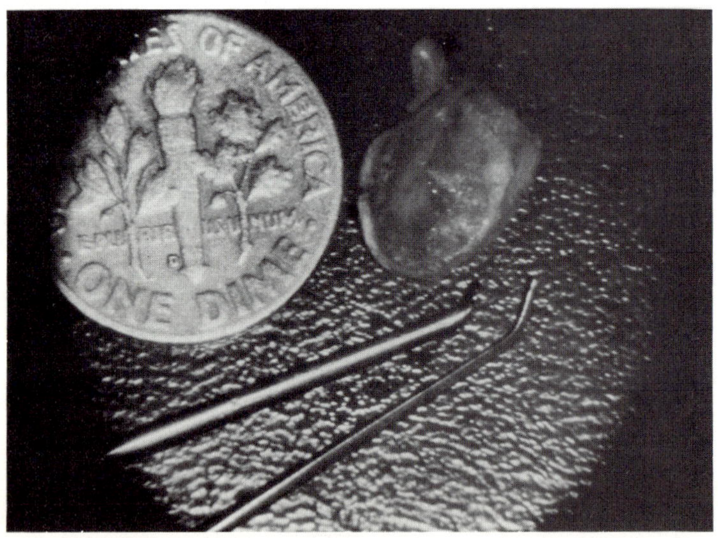

The homographic tympanic membrane and middle ear instruments compared to a dime.

Eardrum transplants are being done in increasing numbers to replace damaged eardrums and middle-ear bones, and to restore loss of hearing caused by infections of the *middle ear* and *mastoid*. They are also being done to repair birth defects of the outer and middle ears.

Dr. Roger E. Wehrs of St. Francis Hospital in Tulsa, Oklahoma, has been working in this field, and he has reported his experiences in transplanting 164 eardrums over a period of three years. He found that well over 90% of the transplants were working well after three years, and that good results have been achieved in seven out of ten ears on which the operation was performed.

Doctor Wehrs' transplanted eardrums were taken from persons who had just died. In some cases, he used the eardrum with attached ear canal skin; in other cases, the eardrum alone; in still others, the eardrum with the *malleus* (hammer) bone attached. Among the cases he helped were people with perforated eardrums, people in whom other eardrum operations had failed, and persons who had had extensive surgery because of mastoid infections.

Ear drums have an advantage over other organ transplants as they are well accepted by the body and do not cause rejection problems that create so much difficulty with heart, liver and kidney transplants.

Dr. Wehrs was able to show, with photographs of healed ears, how the transplants actually became an integral part of the body into which they have been grafted.

The actual procedure during the transplant operation depends on the condition of the ear, and the extent of damage which has to be corrected with the graft. In general, however, only those parts of the eardrum are replaced which are found to be no longer useful. This is why, in some cases, the eardrum alone is used, while in others it is used along with some other parts of the middle ear still attached to it.

11. NEW DRUG DISSOLVES GALLSTONES

THE GALL BLADDER is a pear-shaped organ about four inches long and two inches in diameter. Sometimes, when the gall bladder is diseased, small hard objects form in it. The hard masses, called gallstones, become lodged in the bile duct and can cause much pain.

Researchers at the famous Mayo Clinic, Rochester, Minnesota have succeeded in dissolving gallstones in man—the first time this has been done. So promising are the first results that the National Institute of Arthritis and Metabolic Diseases, which sponsored the Mayo Clinic study, is planning to initiate studies on large numbers of patients.

Little is known about how gallstones are formed, but they are one of the oldest afflictions known to man, and one of the most common. More than 15 million people in America are estimated to have cholesterol gallstones. (Another kind of gallstones, called pigment-stones, occurs mostly in the Eastern part of the world and are uncommon in America.)

In the Mayo Clinic trials, conducted by Dr. Alan F. Hofmann, associate director of the Mayo gastroenterology unit, and by Dr. Johnson L. Thistle, seven women with radiolucent gallstones were given, by mouth, doses of chenodeoxycholic acid (CDC)—the drug that has been found to dissolve them. All seven patients responded favorably to treatment. In four patients the stones have disappeared completely, while in the

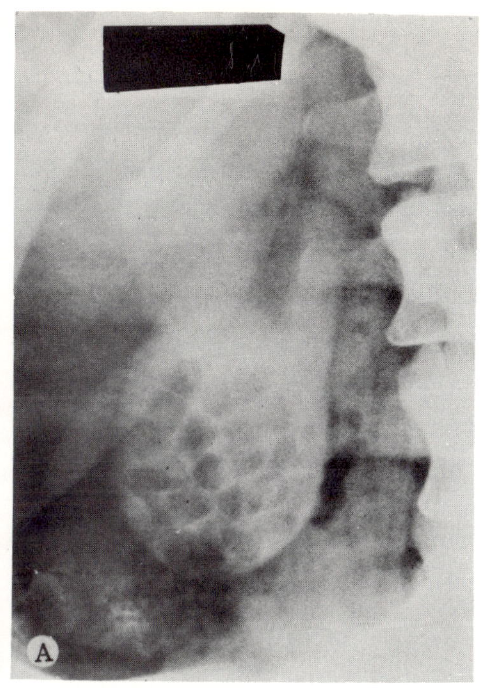

Oral cholecystograms showing multiple stones in a functioning gall bladder (left) and the same stones markedly reduced after 18 months of CDC (below).

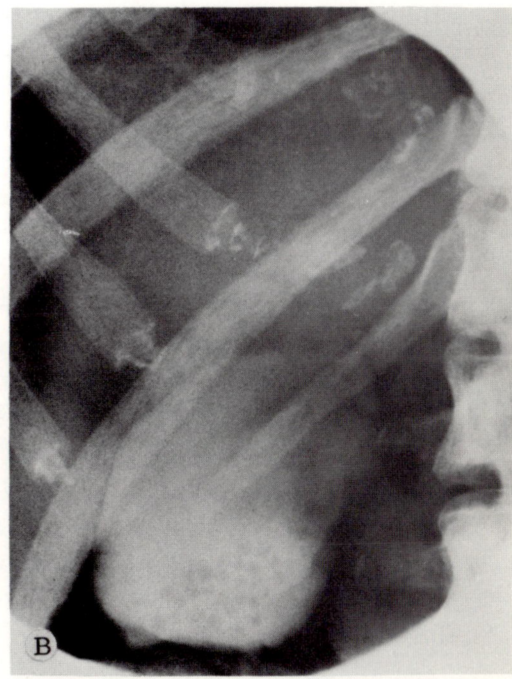

other three women they have become smaller. The treatment has been carried out over a period of two years, and some of the patients whose stones disappeared completely were under treatment for one to two years. Others, in which the stones have diminished, have also been taking CDC over that same long period of time.

The dissolution of the gallstones with CDC is slow, but apparently effective. However, the type of gallstones on which the Mayo team is working is not the kind that suddenly makes a person double up in pain. These are stones that people are not even aware they have. These are called asymptomatic stones, because they cause few or no symptoms which would warn a person who has them that they have formed.

The stones of the Mayo Clinic's patients were discovered during thorough physical examinations at the clinic. Once the stones grow large enough to cause pain, CDC cannot help. Dr. Hofmann says that "by the time many patients find out that they must have something done about their gallstones, then it is too late for our treatment."

The discovery of the dissolving drug could lead to the long-sought method of controlling gallstones without surgery. Obviously, thorough physical examinations will be needed to discover them in order to benefit from the knifeless procedure.

Mayo Clinic is now conducting further trials with CDC, and the preliminary reports of these new tests are also very encouraging. In the latest report, out of 17 new patients receiving CDC, nine were found to have considerably reduced gallstones after the first six months on CDC.

American Indians are particularly susceptible to cholesterol gallstones. As many as 60% to 70% of women in certain tribes develop them. Dr. Thistle thinks that if the larger scale tests prove out, the value of the drug in treatment will be enhanced, and it may be possible to use it as a prophylactic in those high-risk groups.

12. REPAIRING BONES
WITH ELECTRIC CURRENT

TWO PERSONS have already had their bones repaired through the use of electric current; a 14-year-old boy, and a 51-year-old woman. The boy suffered from a rare defect in a leg bone; the woman had fallen down several stairs and had broken her right ankle.

Both repair operations proved that human bones do grow again (regenerate) if electricity is applied to them.

The broken ankle of the woman had refused to heal despite the fact that it was in a cast for 13 weeks. After suffering for a total of two years, she returned to the University of Pennsylvania Hospital where Dr. Carl T. Brighton, director of the Orthopaedic Surgery Research, performed the world's first bone repair operation with electricity.

X-rays of the woman's ankle showed that the fracture was incompletely healed—the right malleolus (the protruding round ankle bone) was loose. Dr. Brighton made a tiny incision in the skin over the loose bone, and inserted a wire cathode into the bone at the point of the fracture. The anode end of the wire was an aluminum grid taped to the skin near-by. The ankle was placed in a cast, and a power-pack consisting of batteries and transistors was attached to the outside of the cast. It was connected to the wires through a "window" in the cast.

Additional material touching on this subject can be found in chapters 18, 23, 26 and 40.

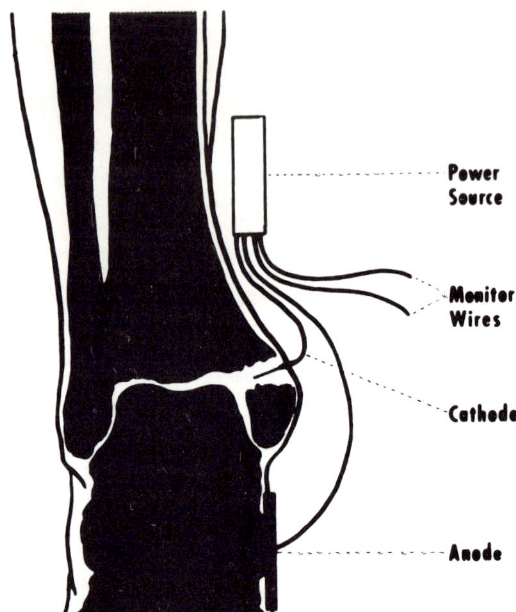

The insertion of the cathode into the non-union
site of a fracture.

Electric current was applied for nine weeks. X-rays then
showed that the break was healed—the bone grew out and
filled in the empty space which was causing the malleolus to
move. The wire was pulled out. She walked on crutches for
two weeks, to "break-in" the new bone joint gently, and then
returned to normal life with the bone perfectly and normally
healed.

In the case of the boy, the bone, instead of being solid all
the way, consisted in part of wobbly cartilage-like material. As
a result, half of the bone on either side of the defect would slip
apart every time the boy would try to stand, and the leg failed
to grow. Technically, the problem was pseudo-arthrosis of the
tibia (main bone of the lower leg).

Doctors at Downstate Medical Center, Brooklyn, New York, implanted electrodes on both sides of the defect and applied current from two D-cell batteries for almost four months. The bone healed.

Researchers working with current bone repairs believe that it can also be used to treat fresh fractures. Animal experiments continue to suggest that the healing time of broken bones may be cut in half by using electricity.

13. NEW CANADIAN DEVICE SOLVES BED-WETTING PROBLEMS

A NEW, CANADIAN-MADE, battery-operated device to help children with a bed-wetting problem, has been approved by the Food and Drug Administration and is now available in this country.

It was designed by a Toronto engineer, Alexander Mozes, who became frustrated because he could not find a method of helping one of his own children.

In its initial testing at the Hospital for Sick Children in Toronto, it has been shown that four out of five bed-wetters can now be relieved of their condition.

According to one of the doctors who carried out that study, no one is quite sure why so many children wet their beds. Yet they do. "I would think about 10% of children have this trouble to some extent," says Dr. James McKendry, a pediatrician who is on the staff of a special clinic for bed-wetters at the hospital. Dr. McKendry says very few bed-wetters have a physical problem, and he admits that he and other physicians are still puzzled about possible psychological reasons.

The new device, called the *Mozes Detector*, wakes the child as soon as he begins to wet. A few drops of urine are enough to activate the detector. This sets off a loud buzzer and at the same time the child feels a small electric impulse—like a tingling—in the groin. This is enough to wake up the child and remind him to go to the bathroom.

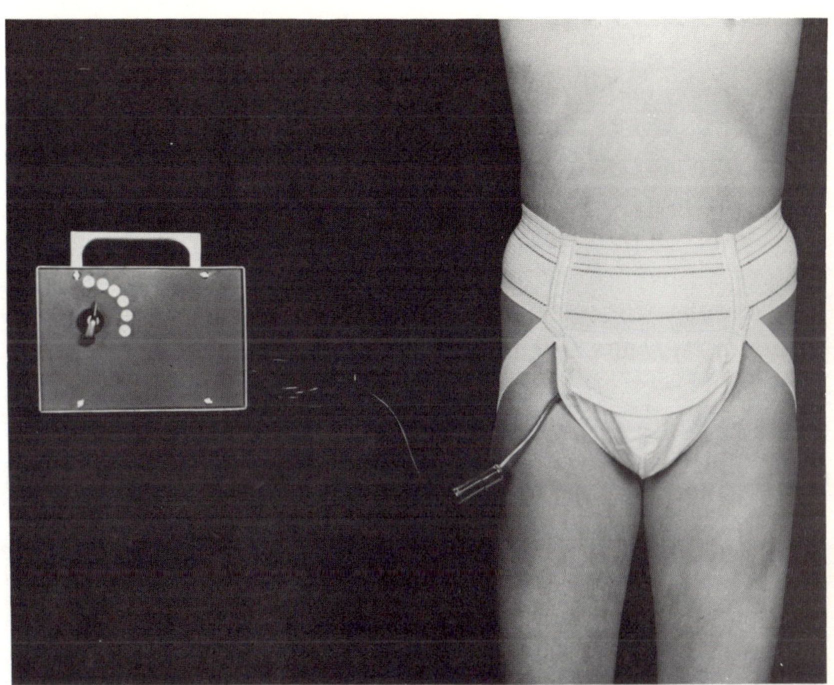

The Mozes Detector worn by a boy.

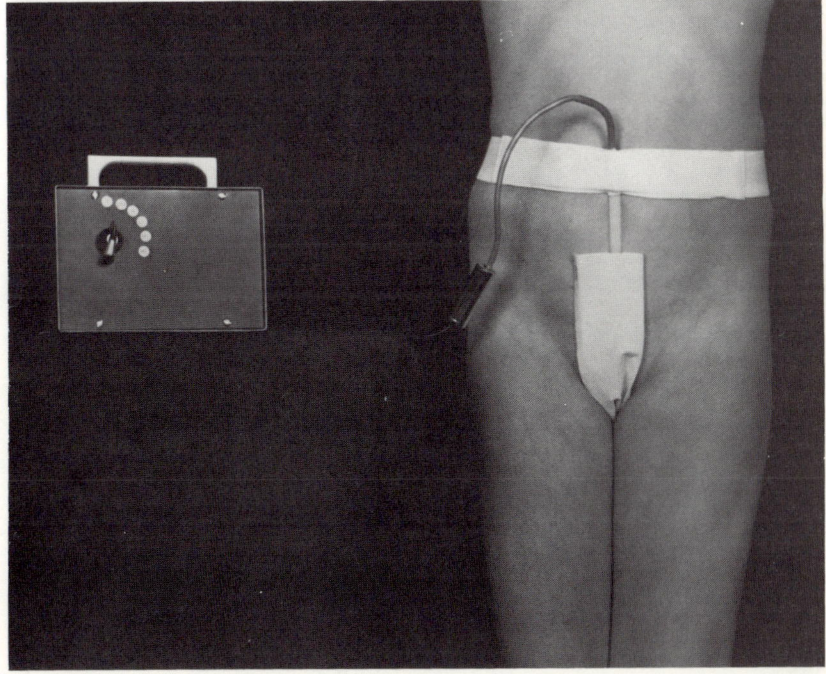

The Mozes Detector worn by a girl.

Another model of the detector, for daytime wear—called the *Mini Model*—has all the components built into a belt worn beneath clothing. In this model, neither the buzzer nor the impulse are shut off until the child stands up.

Doctors report that four out of five children using this detector—even those who were resistant to other methods of treatment—stop wetting in a remarkably short period of time. The average age of the children in the Canadian trials was almost 11 years old. Yet the average treatment time was a mere six and one-half weeks. "This is impressive," says Dr. McKendry.

Writing in a recent issue of the *Canadian Medical Association Journal*, the Toronto pediatrician said the improvement rate of 85% with the Mozes Detector is almost double that of earlier devices which were tested at the clinic.

One of the advantages of the Mozes Detector is that the child never wets the bed. As soon as a few drops of moisture are present, he is awakened. "This was one of the things which frustrated me when I was having a problem with one of my own children," says Mr. Mozes. "The bed had to be pretty wet before the alarm woke the child."

The detector is worn by boys in the form of an athletic-type belt, and by girls in a form closely resembling a sanitary napkin and a belt. The electrodes inside it cannot harm the child. The device itself is operated with ordinary batteries and can be pre-set at various signal strengths as directed by the attending physician. The detector is so designed that it will detect moisture no matter in what position the child sleeps.

The detector can also be used with the buzzer signal only (no electric tingle). The tingle is not used with children under five years of age.

The detector is sold only with a doctor's prescription. Information on the device is available from the Mozes Engineering Ltd., 301 Lesmill Road, Don Mills, Ontario, Canada.

14. RADIOTHERAPY BY REMOTE CONTROL

A NUCLEAR-AGE "HOT ROOM" at New York City's Memorial Hospital is proving valuable in irradiation treatment of tumors in the vagina, nasopharynx (nose) and mouth. It is also being used to treat cancers of the cervix and endometrium (the membrane lining of the uterus).

Conventional radium applications are complicated and time-consuming. They involve a radiation hazard to hospital personnel and, for the patient, necessitate general anesthesia during the insertion of the applicator, followed by a day or two in an isolation room.

The "hot room" removes these difficulties, cuts treatment time from days to minutes, and makes it possible to bombard the tumors with much higher doses of radiation in less time than conventional treatment takes.

The room was developed by Dr. Basil Hilaris and Dr. Ulrich K. Henschke. It consists of a treatment room surrounded by a thick concrete wall, with a control room on the other side of the wall. Communications between the treatment room and the control room are by closed circuit TV and a speaker system. A lead safe in the wall holds the radiation sources—tiny, stainless steel rods containing radioactive cobalt. The rods are welded to the ends of long cables

---

Additional material touching on this subject can be found in chapters 6, 15, 16, 38, 65 and 93.

threaded into flexible plastic tubes, which extend out of the safe into the treatment room.

In actual procedure—to irradiate the vagina, for example—a hollow aluminum applicator is inserted into the vagina and three plastic tubes are connected to it. Then the medical personnel leaves the room. From the control room the three sources of radioactive cobalt are advanced electrically out of the safe, through the plastic tubes, and into the applicator. A sensor inserted in the anus of the patient continuously monitors the treatment to avoid over-irradiation and damage to healthy tissue.

According to Dr. Hilaris, the high-intensity internal radiation made possible by the "hot room," has produced promising results. For example, of thirty-one women who received the treatment prophylactically after surgery for pelvic cancer, there was no tumor recurrence in twenty-seven cases. Promising results are also reported by Dr. Hilaris in treatment for vaginal recurrence of lesions after surgery elsewhere.

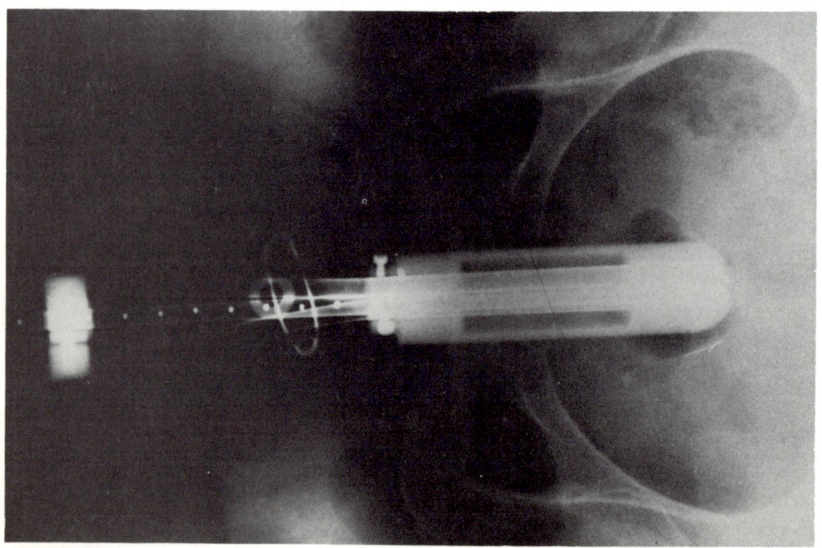

An X-ray photograph showing a vaginal applicator in place.

15. A METHOD OF REMOVING SKIN CANCER BY "SPRAYING"

THOUGH SKIN CANCERS are usually curable in 95% of
the cases, either with irradiation or by surgery, the procedures
have many disadvantages. If the cancers are located in several
places, repeated visits to the doctor are required. If an operation is required, skin grafts are often necessary to repair the
scars left by the removal of the tumors. Skin cancer is also a
typical disease of the aged. Since these patients also suffer
from heart conditions, surgery becomes virtually impossible.

Now, a pioneer in the field of skin cancer cryosurgery, Dr.
Setrag A. Zacarian, director of dermatology at the Springfield
(Mass.) Hospital Medical Center, has developed a technique
for "spraying off" skin cancers with liquid nitrogen.

Dr. Zacarian uses his technique on cancers of the nose, ear,
neck and eyelids, as well as several other areas of the body.
The procedure is simple. He uses a small, hand-held spray unit, of his own design, which is filled with liquid nitrogen.
When he presses the trigger, he releases enough spray to
freeze a skin tumor of almost any size or depth. A thermocou-
ple needle attached to a pyrometer (a special thermometer) is
also inserted into the tumor to measure the temperature. This
is done to make sure that the entire tumor is frozen *inside* to
the degree of coldness required to kill the cancer.

Additional material touching on this subject can be found in chapters 6, 14, 16, 38,
65 and 93.

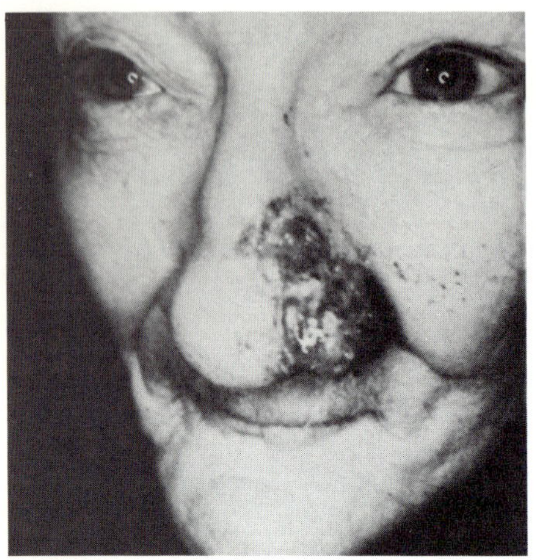

A patient with a large cancer of the nose.

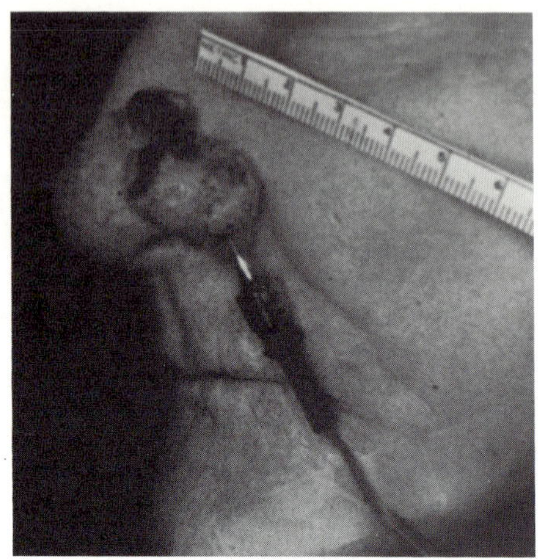

After 3 minutes of freezing with liquid nitrogen, the tumor is reduced.

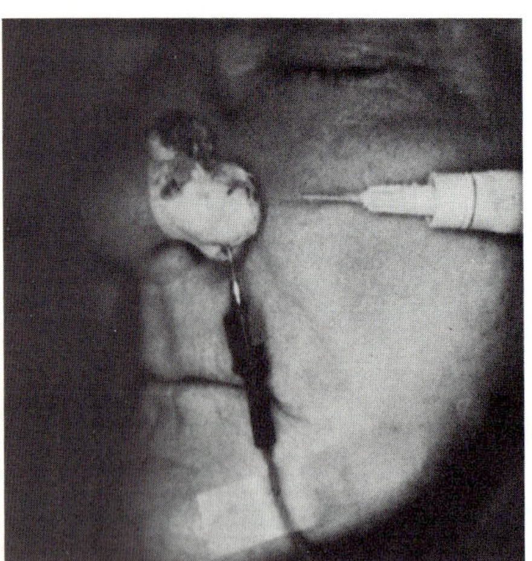

After one week, the tumor begins to slough.

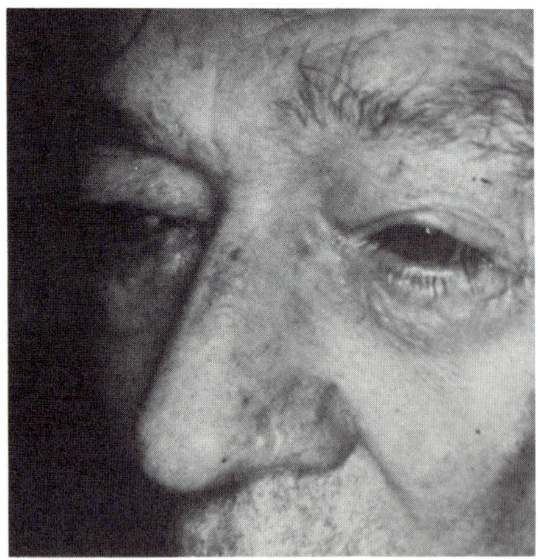

Five weeks after surgery, the tumor is gone.

The correct freezing of the tumor is the most important part of the procedure. Also, not only does the entire tumor have to be deeply frozen inside, it is also necessary to freeze it slightly beyond the visible border to make sure that all the cancerous cells have been killed. This, of course, has to be done with care, in order not to kill healthy tissue. But it must be done, because if all the cancer cells are not frozen dead, the cancer will return. For this reason, Dr. Zacarian considers it essential to monitor the temperature with a pyrometer.

After the tumor is sprayed with liquid nitrogen, a mound-like snowball forms over it for a short period of time. In a few hours, the area blisters and turns red. Shortly thereafter, a scab starts to form, and within a week the tumor begins to slough off. After a month, it has disappeared and the skin is healed and smooth.

The entire operation which takes three or four minutes, requires no anesthesia and leaves minimal scars. Consequently, there is no need for skin grafts.

In the past eight years, Dr. Zacarian has treated 1,792 skin cancers with cryosurgery and has achieved a cure rate of 97%. About three in 100 patients had a recurrence of the cancer within six months to five years.

Dr. Zacarian is extremely confident of the value of cryosurgery in the treatment of skin cancer and believes it can be effective in all forms of skin cancer except when the tumor is exceptionally large and conventional surgery would be indicated. But these cases are extremely rare.

16. CRYOSURGERY
FOR MOUTH CANCERS

MANY CANCERS of the mouth are quick killers. Once having reached an advanced stage, they cannot be operated on. The bulky, bleeding and foul-smelling tumors in the mouth or in the throat are very painful and, in many cases, nothing can be done for the incurable patient except keeping him "doped" with morphine until he dies.

Now, hope is on the horizon for the sufferers from these formerly incurable cancers, particularly from the cancers of the tonsil, palate, pharynx and the soft tissues in the mouth.

Dr. J. Ryan Chandler, professor and chairman of the Department of Otolaryngology at the University of Miami School of Medicine has reported on the use of cryosurgery. In cryosurgery the area is frozen with liquid nitrogen applied through a crochet needle-like probe. The test was made on 64 patients who were considered inoperable and incurable. In addition, after the first results were in, 11 more persons were treated with cryosurgery as the initial cure for their cancers.

Of the 64 patients, 37 were treated for recurrent cancers in the mouth. These were persons who were previously treated with radiation or who had surgery, but in whom the cancers reappeared. Dr. Chandler's overall success rate was about 50%.

Additional material touching on this subject can be found in chapters 6, 14, 15, 16, 38, 65 and 68.

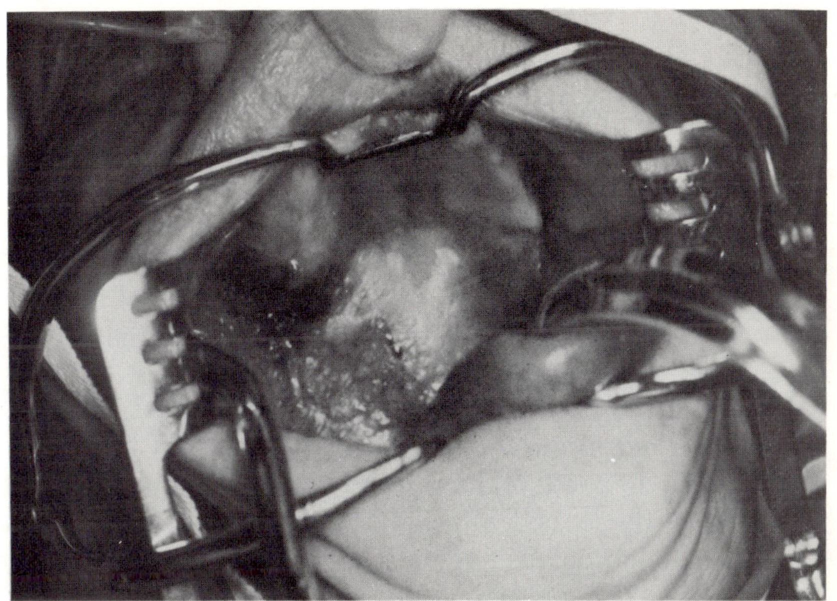

Infiltrative cancer of the mouth.

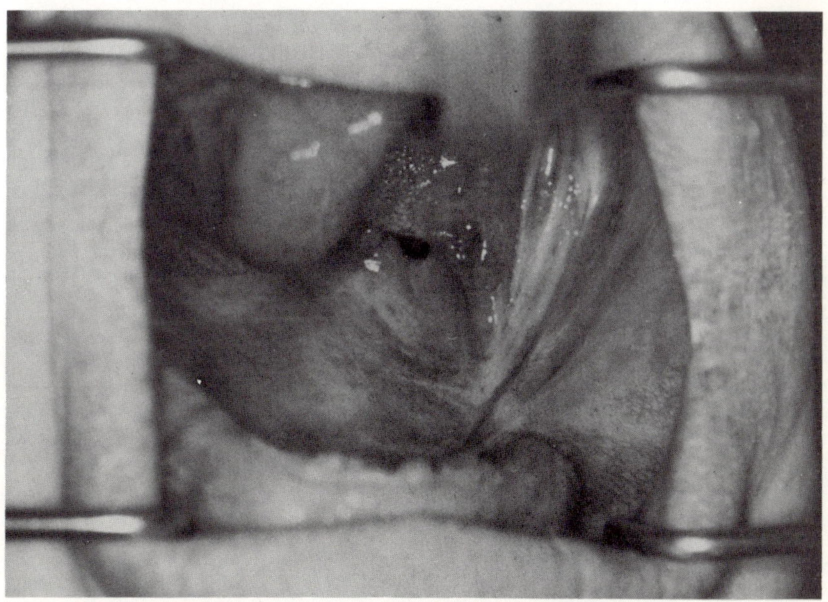

Cancers of the mouth shown above, one and one-half years after treatment.

Of the 37 patients treated for the mouth cancers, 16 were saved. At the time this is being written, seven survivors are within the first year of treatment and the other nine have passed the one year mark. One is alive and well three years after the surgery.

Dr. Chandler's technique in treating the terminal cases (patients who are dying) is very aggressive. The tip of the ice probe is carried right next to arteries to make sure that all of the cancer tumor is frozen dead. If bleeding results, it is taken care of after the freezing. After cryosurgery, there is a great deal of swelling inside the mouth, and to prevent a patient from choking to death, a tracheotomy (tube insertion into the throat from the outside to allow breathing) is performed before the operation. This is major surgery and it carries with it all the dangers of major surgery, but according to Dr. Chandler it can result in some cures in otherwise incurable patients.

Dr. Chandler's experience with the survival-technique and the initial cure obtained in nine of 11 patients leads him to comment that we now have not only a permanent addition to the methods of treating cancer of the head and neck, but that with some more experience it might become "the initial treatment of choice for some patients with carcinomas and other malignant neoplasms of the tonsil, pharynx and buccal mucosa."

At present Dr. Chandler is using the new technique only on selected patients.

17. NEW X-RAY SYSTEM TO INVESTIGATE BRAIN DISEASES

A UNIQUE COMPUTER-AIDED X-ray unit, hailed as one of the greatest X-ray technique improvements, has been developed in England. The unit, called the Emi-Scanner, is in operation at Atkinson Morley's Hospital in Wimbledon, England, and installations have been ordered by several Canadian and American institutions, including the Mayo Clinic and the Massachusetts General Hospital.

The Emi-Scanner was developed by a British engineer, Godfrey Hounsfield, and its development won Mr. Hounsfield the coveted British MacRobert Award. This award, often described as the Nobel Prize for engineering, consists of a Gold Medal and $60,000 in prize money.

The Emi-Scanner is used only for brain examinations: in the investigation of brain diseases, such as tumors, cysts and hemorrhages.

Conventional X-ray pictures have an important inherent fault: they show a three-dimensional object in a two-dimensional picture without perspective. This often confuses the information shown on the picture. Also, details of brain tissue are masked in X-ray pictures by the surrounding, denser bone of the skull. The Emi system overcomes these obstacles, and also makes unnecessary anesthesias and injections of air or opaque fluids into the brain. Such procedures

Additional material touching on this subject can be found in chapters 94 and 98.

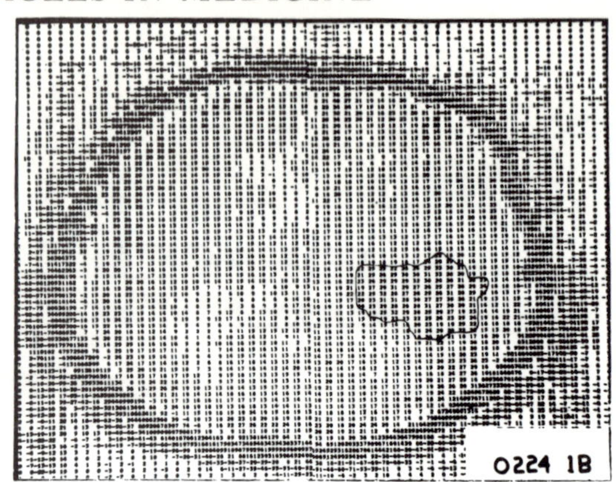

An Emi-Scanner computer print-out showing a primary intercerebral hemorrhage.

are often required with conventional X-ray brain studies, and they are not without risk to the patient.

With the new system, the patient is inconvenienced no more than by a chest X-ray, and 100 times more information on brain tissue is extracted from the X-rays than is possible with conventional techniques. The scanning procedure, which does not even involve taking off one's street clothing, takes only 4½ minutes.

The technique, called *computerized transverse axial tomography*, involves scanning the patient's brain with very sensitive X-ray detectors, while the scanning unit is being rotated around the patient's head. In a 4½ minute period of time, the scanner makes 28,800 readings of the brain. The information is fed to a small computer which reproduces a picture of the brain on a display screen. The picture is extremely detailed—it consists of 6,400 picture points, each representing the X-ray absorption of the tissue of the brain in that spot.

The doctor can examine the picture on the screen, or have it photographed for future reference. The computer can also print out the information in a pattern of numbers, giving accurate and detailed information on the brain tissue at each point in the patient's head.

18. CERAMICS SHORE
UP BAD BONES

ONE OF THE oldest machines, the wedge, and one of the oldest materials, ceramics, have been combined by Doctors William B. Campbell and Edward J. Eyring of Ohio State University's Bio-Medical Engineering Center, Columbus, Ohio, to provide an improved surgical technique for straightening, lengthening and correcting angular deformities (bent bones) of legs, hips, arms, fingers, and feet. The operation is called *open wedge osteotomy*, and has been an accepted surgical procedure for many years.

In this procedure, for example, to straighten out a bent bone, the bone is broken (under general anesthesia) and repositioned correctly with the wedge holding it in place. The wedge must hold the broken ends of the bone apart, and in position, until the space is filled in by growing bone as the area heals.

The conventional wedge made of bone has several limitations. For example, it must be obtained and shaped at the time of surgery. The results obtained with bone wedges are uncertain as all bone wedges shrink somewhat after being grafted in position.

Dr. Campbell developed the ceramic wedge to eliminate the shortcomings of the bone wedges and to shorten the time

---

Additional material touching on this subject can be found in chapters 6, 12, 26 and 40.

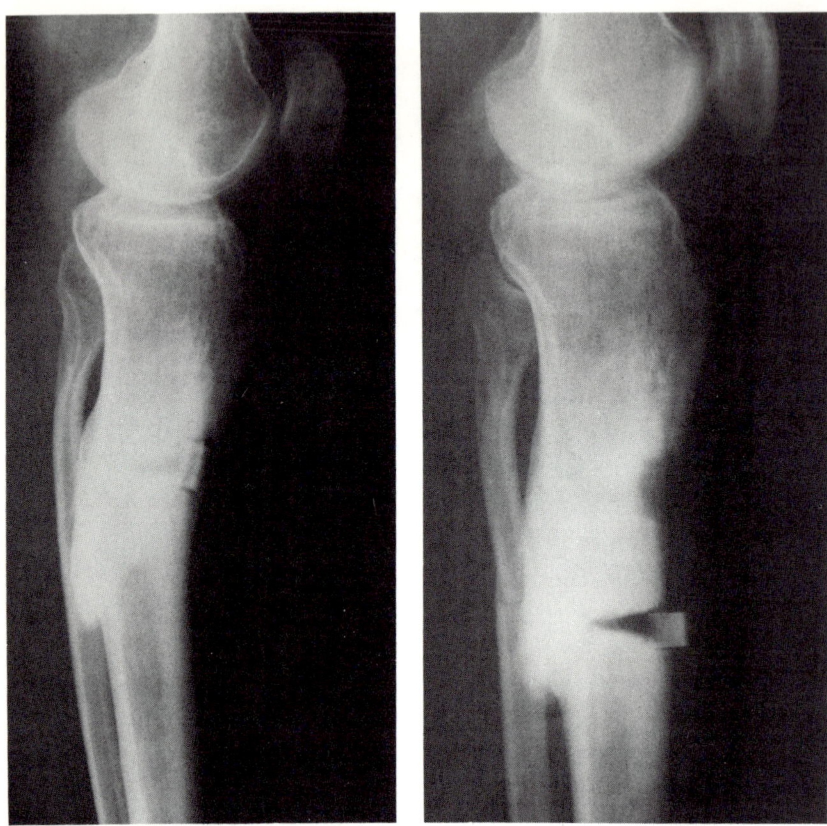

The repair of a badly healed old fracture, near the knee. In the photo to the left, the tibia has been broken and a ceramic wedge inserted to partially straighten it. To the right, the bone has been broken again and a second wedge inserted below the first one.

required for the surgery. The pure, white ceramic wedge is made of aluminum oxide, a cheap, common material used in production of synthetic gem stones. It is chemically inert in the human body (causes no chemical reaction in the body) and is well accepted by the living tissue (it may be left in place after the bone fills in).

The ceramic is stronger than human bone and contibutes to much earlier recoveries. In some cases hospital stays have been reduced from 30 days to three days.

The size and the shape of the ceramic wedge that may be needed for a given operation can be determined by doctors from X-rays taken before the surgery. The wedge is then made to order in the laboratory, and is ready for insertion at the time of surgery.

Some 40 patients have had the new wedges inserted during operations performed at the university's hospital. The patients have ranged in age from six months to 46 years. The results have been excellent.

19. REBUILDING THE BATTERED KNEE

THERE WAS A TIME when, if an athlete suffered a serious knee injury, his career was finished. In recent years, we have made great strides in understanding the various types of injury that occur, and methods of repair have been developing in giant steps.

The amount of leisure time an individual has today is constantly increasing, and as a result more and more people are actively participating in sports. Consequently the number of injuries has increased. This, in turn, triggered a concerted effort by orthopedic surgeons to find newer and more effective methods of treatment.

One area that has been of particular concern to orthopedists is the knee; especially where there is any device connected to the leg which prevents full motion of the knee. These include spikes on baseball shoes, cleats on football shoes, roller skates, ice-skates, and skis. With sudden twisting action and body contact, the knee can be injured seriously and frequently.

The most common injuries are sprains of the ligaments and torn menisci. (Meniscus is a discoid shaped movable cartilage in the knee joint.) These usually respond well to rest and splinting for the sprains and removal of the meniscus when it is torn.

Additional material touching on this subject can be found in chapter 33.

When a person suffers combined injuries of the knee, that is, when he tears the meniscus plus neighboring ligaments, repair is usually a must. Once, doctors would simply rest these injuries, either by using elastic bandages or a plaster cast. Today, surgery has been found to yield the best and quickest results in returning the athlete to action.

The new orthopedic procedures are not limited to the sports injuries. As Dr. William A. Liebler, an orthopedic surgeon at Lenox Hill Hospital in New York City, and orthopedist to the New York Rangers hockey squad, points out, "It doesn't matter if the patient is a football player or a businessman.   If he tears the knee ligament in a flying tackle or running for a commuter train, the resultant injuries are the same."

The big difference, of course, between an athlete and a businessman is that the athlete is usually in better physical shape, and will heal much sooner. A second factor pointed out by Dr. Liebler is that the athlete is better motivated to recover since his career is at stake. As a result, he is likely to get better faster.

A common injury in football is a combination of torn meniscus and two ligaments, called the anterior cruciate ligament and the medial collateral ligament. This injury causes instability, and if not repaired, the player permanently loses his stability and hence, his power and agility.

This particular injury has been under study by Dr. James Nicholas and his group at the Institute for Sports Medicine and Athletic Trauma at Lenox Hill Hospital, New York City, for the past 10 years.

From this study, a method of treatment has evolved making it possible today to treat serious injuries successfully. The main finding of the study is that, if the direction of force on the knee could be reversed and the appropriate damaged structures in it repaired, this would result in a stable knee.

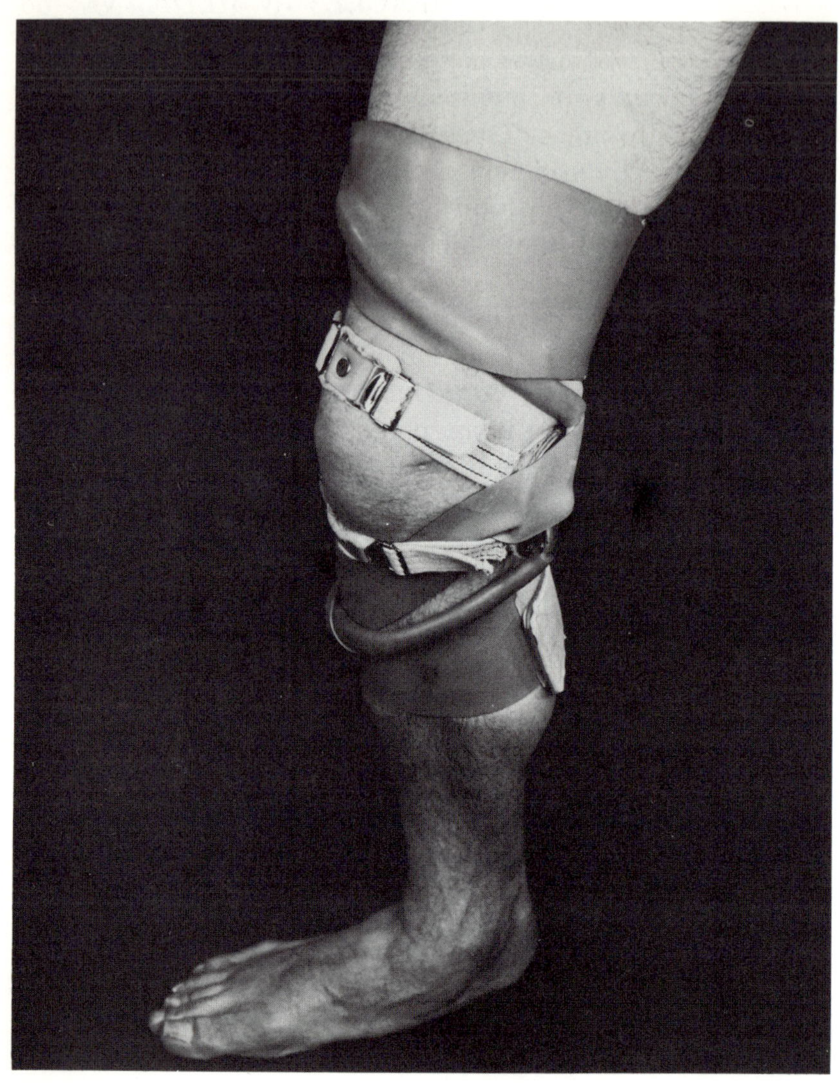

A Lenox Hill Derotation Brace.

(Reversing the direction of force means putting the knee back in the position it was in before the injury. For example, if the knee was hit from the outside inwards, it has to be pushed in the direction from which it was hit.)

From this, a surgical technique developed—the so-called "5-in-1." This is a knee stabilization operation which involves stapling torn knee ligaments to the bone and which consists of five operative steps. The "5-in-1" goes hand in hand with a special brace which is fitted before the operation and applied after six weeks in a cast. The procedure also includes a prompt, active exercise program. Usually, within three months, the knee is stable enough to start using it.

The special brace—called the Lenox Hill Derotation Brace —was devised only a few years ago by the Lenox Hill Brace Shop in New York. It is custom made and is remarkably effective as an excellent safeguard against knee injuries. Eventually, it may become standard athletic equipment to be worn by all players.

One does not have to be operated on in order to benefit from it. "The brace," reports Dr. Liebler, "is found to be enough to stabilize the knee if the injury was not too severe, as with Brad Park. He did not have the operation but was able to finish out the season with the brace. Many athletes have finished out a season with the use of the brace. After the season, the knee is repaired and the athlete is ready to start a new season with a stable knee." Joe Namath, and many other top athletes have benefited from the "5-in-1" and brace combination.

20. AUSTRALIAN INVENTION HELPS REMEDY CURVATURE OF SPINE

AN AUSTRALIAN ENGINEER has designed equipment which allows surgeons to correct many cases of curvature of the spine.

The equipment, now widely used in this country and in Canada, was developed by Mr. Arthur Sherwood, associate professor of bio-mechanics at the University of Sydney in conjunction with Dr. Allan Frederick Dwyer, an orthopedic surgeon of Sydney's Mater Misericordiae Hospital.

The equipment consists of a series of titanium screws which surgeons implant in the vertebrae of patients. A titanium cable is passed through the screw heads and tightened with a special cable tensioner to straighten the curve in the spine. Called the Dwyer-Sherwood technique, the operation is done to help persons with scoliosis, or curvature of the spine.

Persons with scoliosis have an S-shaped spine, with one main curve and a smaller curve in the opposite direction. The Dwyer-Sherwood technique is used to correct the curve in the lower spine whenever that curve is convex (in the shape of the lower half of the S).

In the actual operation, one rib is removed, to give the surgeon room to work. The screws are then set into the front of the vertebrae, inside the rib cage. The cable—which is made of seven strands, each made of 19 titanium wires—is fed through holes in the screw heads once the screws are in place.

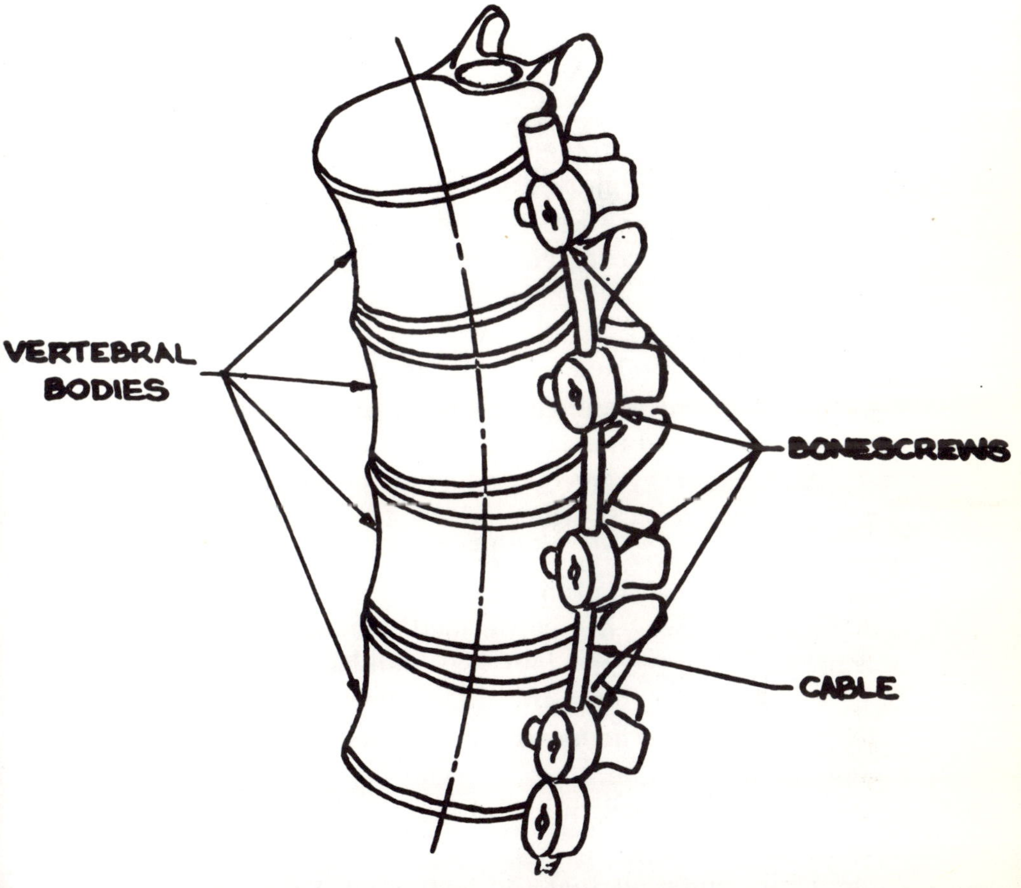

A sketch showing how the Dwyer-Sherwood spinal fusion system works.

The cable is then tightened, one screw at a time, with the cable tensioner, aligning the vertebrae with each other in a straight line. The tensioner is equipped with a spring gauge for measuring tension. Another tool—called a modified mechanical crimper—is used to close the screw head holes over the cable and hold it securely in place.

Mr. Sherwood also developed anchorage plates to give the

bone screws (which act like washers) a firm hold in all vertebrae, and it is now common practice for the surgeons to use these plates on all vertebrae along the curvature.

The Dwyer-Sherwood method allows the surgeon to remove discs from the spine in the affected area. Also, it keeps the spine straight while the vertebrae fuse together in the affected section after these discs have been removed. After the discs have been removed, the rib that was removed is cut up into small pieces, and these are inserted into the disc space as a bone graft to aid in the fusing of the spine.

The process can take a few months, and when completed, the implanted screws and cable can be removed. In practice, since the screws and the cable have so far not caused trouble in any patients, they are being left in the body.

One American institution, where the operation is performed frequently, is the children's hospital of the Harvard Medical School, in Boston. Dr. John E. Hall, its chief of orthopedic surgery, has performed almost 100 of these operations during the past four years and has been impressed, as he put it, "with their efficacy in selected cases."

Dr. Hall says that he has been extremely pleased with this ingenious device, because it enables him to "manage problems which had no real good answer before its development."

Dr. Hall points out that the technique is particularly indicated in a child who has scoliosis associated with myelomeningocele (spina bifida with both spinal cord and its membranes protruding from the spine) and in whom the back of the spine is grossly abnormal.

21. NEW TOOL TO FIGHT BLINDNESS

HOPE SHINES BRIGHT for victims of *diabetic retinopathy*, a condition responsible for the causing of blindness in over 150,000 people now living in the United States.

In diabetic retinopathy and certain other eye conditions (for example, a cataract caused by being hit in the eye with a baseball), the vitreous (jelly-like) substance in the eye is often clouded because of repeated bleedings. Or, it may form strands, pulling on the retina and causing detachment of the retina. (The *retina* is an inner skin of the eyeball which envelops the jelly-like tissue.) Vision is badly impaired.

Doctors are optimistic that a new operation called *vitrectomy* may improve the condition of these sufferers, and may also help many blinded by other diseases.

To perfect the new operation, a new surgical tool, the *vitreous infusion cutter* (VISC), was created by a team of bio-medical engineers.

Prior to the invention of VISC, surgeons had to attempt a complicated operation to help victims regain some vision. The eye had to be entered from the front, which required the removal of the cornea and the lens. Using VISC, the eye is entered from the side, away from the delicate parts in the front. The incision is tiny.

Additional material touching on this subject can be found in chapters 9, 25, 30, 36, 56 and 70.

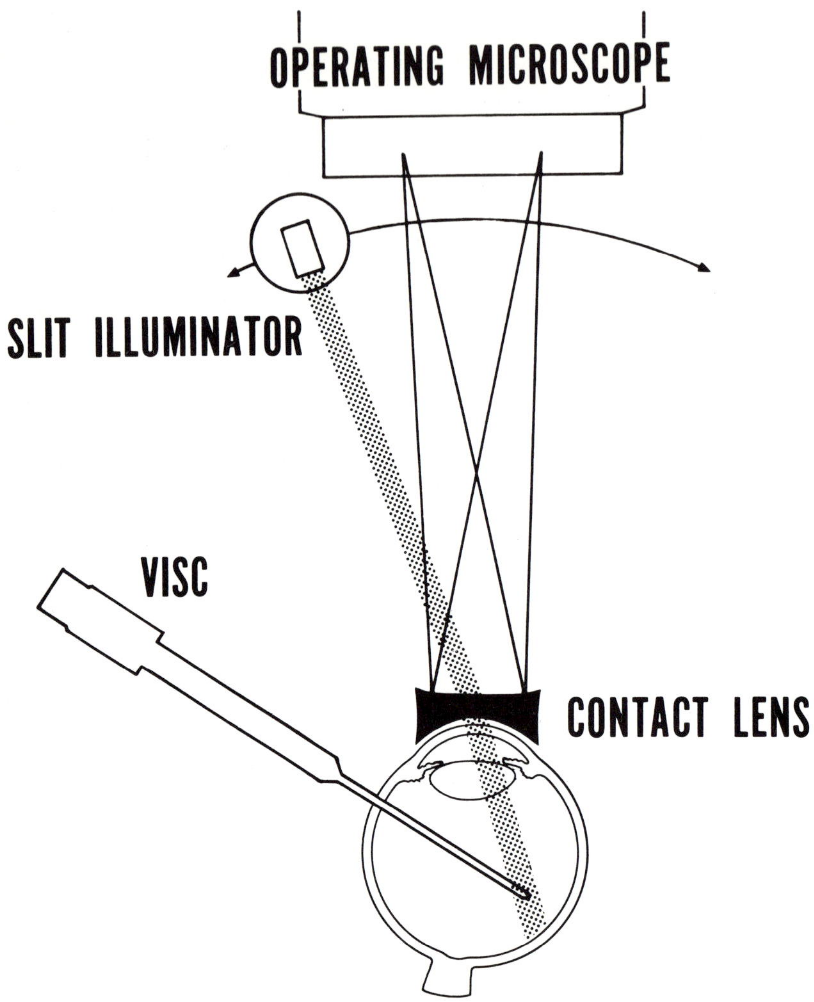

A contact lens on the surface of the eye magnifies the light projected into the eyeball while the operating microscope helps the surgeon observe his progress. Note how the instrument enters the eye from the side, away from the delicate parts in the front.

VISC consists of a small rotary knife driven by a motor, a suction system to suck out and remove the diseased jelly-like tissue, and an injection system to refill the cavity with a saline solution. (The body slowly absorbs the saline solution and replaces it with normal eye fluid.)

The operation is performed under a special automated operating microscope equipped with a light which always illuminates the operating area. The rotating edge of the VISC knife allows the surgeon to cut the tissue to be removed. Simultaneously with the cutting, the suction mechanism removes the diseased tissue and the injection unit constantly drips the appropriate amount of the saline solution into the eyeball. When the operation is over, the VISC is withdrawn and the tiny cut stitched closed.

Vitrectomy was developed by doctors Robert Machemer, Helmut Buettner, Edward W. D. Norton, and bio-engineer Jean-Marie Parel of the Bascom Palmer Eye Institute of the University of Miami, Florida.

Surgeons at the Bascom Palmer Eye Institute have performed over 150 vitrectomies, improving or restoring vision in patients whose eyes were considered untreatable before vitrectomy was developed.

A fully automated, surgical microscope for routine use in this operation has been set up in the Veterans Administration hospital in Miami, Florida. In general, however, there is still a shortage of both the new cutters and the special microscopes, and the number of operations by eye specialists trained to perform the new operation is greatly limited.

22. HEALTH PILLOW
RELIEVES BREATHING DIFFICULTIES

AN AUSTRALIAN HOUSEWIFE, Mrs. Josephine Zaghini, accidentally invented a special health pillow when she decided to find out why her son Anthony, 16, was disturbed in his sleep by sinusitis attacks.

Apparently, when he was sleeping on his side, the pillow bunched around his face making breathing difficult. "He

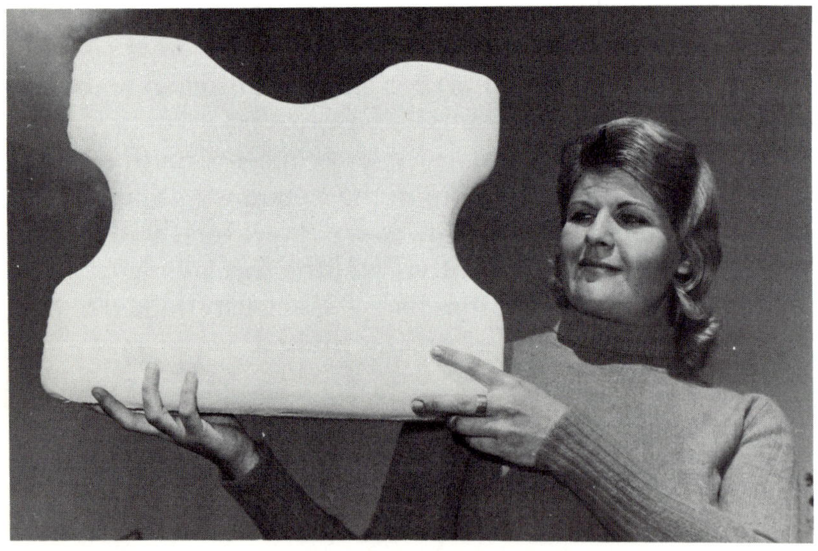

The Australian Bellacomfort health pillow.

Additional material touching on this subject can be found in chapter 89.

seemed to be punching his pillow continually in an effort to make indentations around his nose and mouth," Mrs. Zaghini said. "I made semi-circular cut-outs in a piece of foam rubber, and he was able to sleep easier almost immediately."

Mrs. Zaghini gradually improved the design, and now her patented pillow is available in proper sizes for adults, children and babies. The adult pillow is a 24 inch by 16 inch by 5 inch piece of non-crease foam rubber with semi-circular cut-outs on three sides. One cut-out is for the neck and shoulder, and the other two allow the nose and mouth to "overhang" the actual pillow without obstruction while still supporting the jaw and cheek-bone.

In medical applications, a receptacle for nose or mouth discharge can be easily placed in the side cut-outs. It is claimed that the pillow aids persons with breathing problems, particularly those suffering from asthma, hay fever, and from various sinus problems.

Mrs. Zaghini found that the pillow also appeals to women as a beauty aid. "Women today spend a lot of money on face creams to prevent lines and wrinkles," she said. "Yet every night they bury their faces in pillows, subjecting the skin to hours of distortion.

"Just think of how many mornings you wake up with lines etched on your skin because of a wrinkle or crease in the pillow."

In Australia, an adult-size pillow sells for about six dollars. Inquiries about the pillow may be sent to Mrs. Josephine Zaghini, Ingham, Queensland 4850, Australia.

23. HOW SHORT PEOPLE CAN BECOME TALLER

A GERMAN DEVICE is making short people taller—from the inside. Called the *Kuentscher distancing pin*, it's a stainless steel splint, or pin, with a "bump."

Here is how it works: the thigh bone is severed with an *internal saw* invented by Dr. Gerhard Kuentscher, world-famous German bone surgeon. The saw is inserted from the end of the bone (see photo), making it unnecessary to cut open the thigh. Then the "bump" of the splint is fitted between the two ends of the bone, keeping them apart. The distance between the two ends is no more than an inch and a quarter. Later, new bone grows out and fills in the gap, making the patient an inch or so taller.

New bone could grow over a greater distance than an inch and a quarter, but this would mean too much stretch for nerves and arteries. If necessary, the bone can be lengthened again in a second operation, sometime after the first has healed. At this point the nerves and arteries will have adjusted to the new length.

Patients can walk and return to work or school a week after the operation. When the bone is firm enough, the pin can be removed.

The new distancing pin is also expected to be of great help in cases in which a person has suffered a serious multiple fracture of the *femur* (thigh bone). This often happens in high

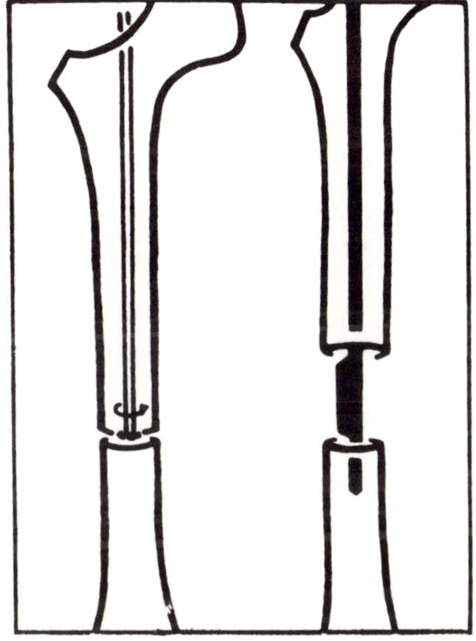

In order to lengthen the leg, an internal saw saws from within (left), making it unnecessary to cut open the thigh. The saw is then replaced by a distancing pin (right) which keeps the stumps apart.

speed car collisions in which the bone is often shattered into many small pieces.

Until now, the shattered bone was pieced together by the use of casts or Thomas splint appliances, and at least three months was required before doctors could determine whether the bone was actually healing again. As a result of this operation, even when successful, the shattered bone was shorter than before. The end result was that one leg became shorter than the other, creating harmful changes in the spine.

With the use of the new distancing pin, a broken bone is splinted from the inside with pins, and the patient can walk again in one week.

A special center for these pin operations has been set up at Bevensen Hospital, Hamburg, West Germany. In charge of the splint operations is Dr. Siegfried Fischer, who invented the distancing pin together with Dr. Kuentscher.

24. PORTABLE CORONARY ALARM WARNS OF IMPENDING ATTACKS

HEART PATIENTS can now receive advance warning of impending trouble from a pocket-size electronic monitor, which can save their lives!

Called VIDA (for **V**entricular **I**mpulse **D**etector and **A**larm), the monitor weighs less than five ounces, including battery, and is connected to the chest by two pasted-on electrodes. The device can be worn in the shirt pocket, on a belt, or under clothing, and occupies about as much room as 1 ½ decks of cards.

VIDA automatically detects irregular heartbeats, and instantly sounds a warning buzz. The wearer can then call his doctor, hold the phone up to the monitor, and transmit his electrocardiogram to a special receiver in the doctor's office for quick analysis and medical advice.

Sudden deaths from heart attacks claim 650,000 lives in this country each year. Most sudden cardiac deaths are caused by a change in heart rhythm called *ventricular fibrillation*. Ventricular fibrillation prevents the heart from pumping blood. If uncorrected, it can cause death within a minute or two. It is generally agreed by leading cardiologists that the symptoms of a heart attack most always develop at least two to three hours before a death-dealing attack. The VIDA device is intended to warn of impending ventricular fibrillation.

Additional material touching on this subject can be found in chapters 7, 32, 84, 94, 96 and 99.

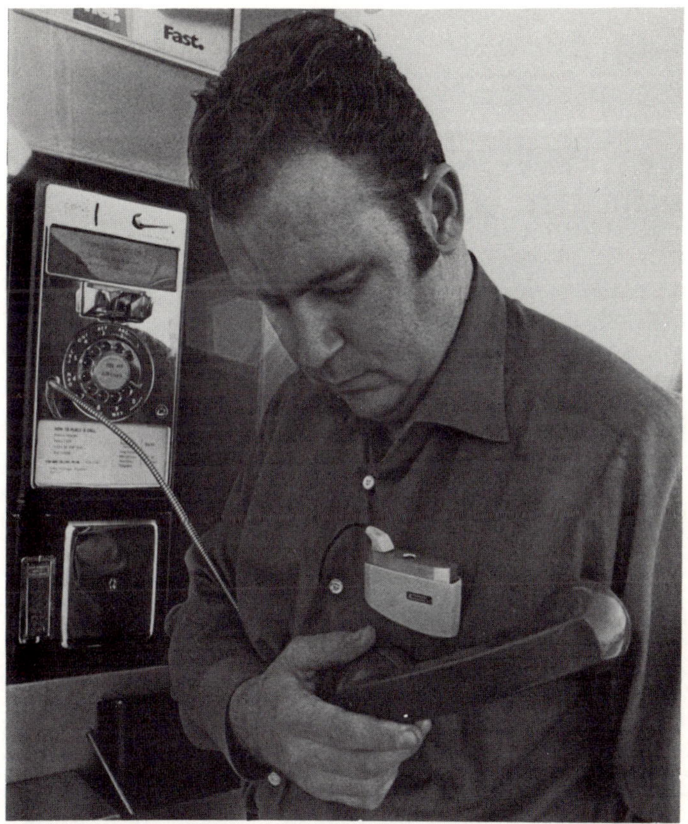

To transmit the ECG over the telephone, the user simply places the telephone mouthpiece against the VIDA monitor.

Potential users of the VIDA monitor are persons who have already suffered one heart attack, or have experienced occasional heart rhythm abnormalities. It is also of potential value to those who have a very high risk of heart attack due to cigarette smoking, high blood pressure and high levels of fat and cholesterol in their blood.

The device was developed by Dr. John W. Gofman, a well-known California cardiologist, and the 1972 co-recipient of the $50,000 Stouffer Prize for outstanding research on heart disease. His co-developer is engineer Robert L. Chapman.

25. NEW TYPEWRITER
FOR THE HANDICAPPED

IF YOU CAN MOVE no other part of your body than your head, you can type with this British-invented "Finger of Light."

Handicapped persons, including those completely paralyzed except for a five degree head movement, can easily learn to operate this PILOT (**P**atient **I**nitiated **L**ight **O**perated **T**ele-control) typewriter system consisting of an electric typewriter, a headband mounted light unit, and a keyboard of photo-electric cells.

The keyboard is laid out in a standard typewriter keyboard pattern. Beneath each symbol appearing on the keyboard is a small hole containing a photoelectric-cell. To type a symbol, the person fixes his "finger of light" on the hole beneath the symbol. This triggers a switch on the special typewriter, causing it to type out the same symbol on which the beam of light is focused.

The "finger of light" is a beam from a light unit attached to a specially designed headband fitted to the crown of the person's head. (The light unit can also be affixed to the handicapped person's eyeglasses.) If the doctor should decide that the patient cannot wear the head-mounted light unit, the unit can be modified to be attached to the hand.

An important feature of this system is its three-speed delay mechanism adjustable to the typist's speed and proficiency.

Additional material touching on this subject can be found in chapter 30.

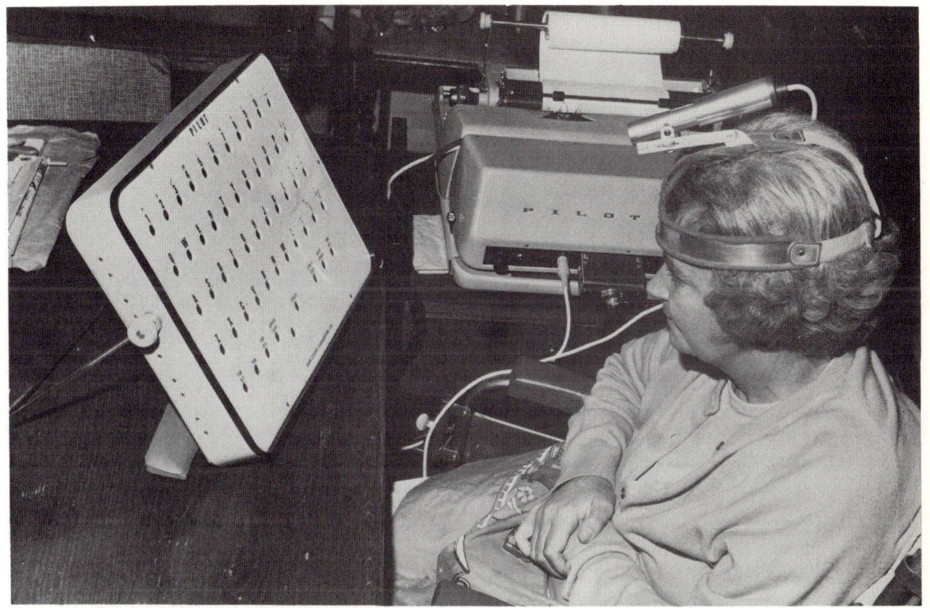

A woman suffering from syringomelia writing a book with the aid of a PILOT typewriter.

The speeds can be set to allow for a learning period, and can be adjusted to handle a more proficient typing operation, and also a normally accepted commercial speed. This is accomplished by a "time-lag" which regulates the amount of time between the striking of the symbol of the light beam and the actual typing motion of the typewriter.

At the slower speeds, the light must rest on the symbol for a while, while at the high speed it needs merely to flash on it. This allows the beginner to familiarize himself with the keyboard and minimize the possibility of striking by accident unwanted symbols as he searches the board for the required symbol.

The PILOT system is manufactured in England by Hugh Steeper Ltd., of Queen Mary's Hospital in London. It is available in the U.S. through S. H. Camp & Co., Jackson, Michigan 49204. The price ranges from $1,600 to $2,000.

26. NEW IMPLANT MATERIAL
FOR ORTHOPEDICS AND ORAL SURGERY

A BRAND-NEW MATERIAL for implants in orthopedics
and reconstructive surgery has been developed by Dr. Charles
A. Humsy, a chemical engineer at the Fondern Orthopedic
Center of the Methodist Hospital in Houston, Texas.

Dr. Humsy says the material, which will probably be called
Proplast, is "probably the first material that has been
designed from the ground up for use in the body."

The new material is a porous, felt-like composite of *Teflon*
and space-age supercarbons. Its rough surface allows tissue to
grow into it, leading to good stability of the implant made out
of it. The body does not reject it. It can be used for coating
other materials and it can also be made up in a block and
carved to shape.

Extensive experiments are now being conducted with
animals to see how the material can be used in the future.
One possibility is artificial tendons. Dr. Frederick B. Kessler,
director of the hand clinic at the Ben Taub General Hospital,
has tried it on several patients, but the results have been in-
conclusive.

The longest experience with Proplast in humans is over
two-and-a-half years. The material was used to make a new

Additional material touching on this subject can be found in chapters 18, 40 and
81.

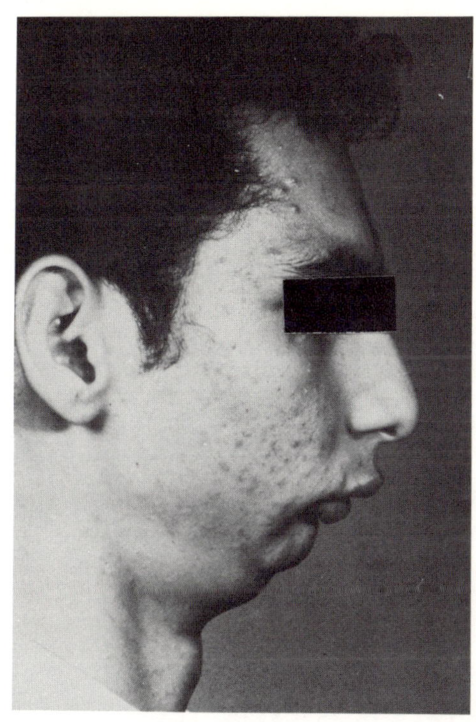

A patient with a "bird chin" before his corrective operation (left) and after (below).

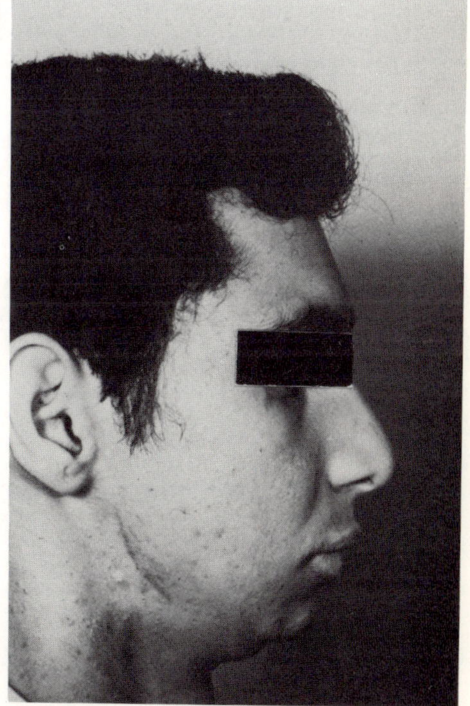

temporo-mandibular joint. This is the joint in the mouth which controls the movement of the lower jaws.

The patient was a young man who suffered from ankylosis —"frozen jaw." It started soon after his birth and at the age of eight he couldn't move his lower jaw. He was operated on to "free" the jaw—a complex operation in which Teflon sheets were placed over the stumps of the joint to allow it to "slide" and move. This helped for a few years—then the jaw froze again.

It was impossible to repair the jaw because a regular metal condyle—a long bone with a "hook"—screwed into the bone will not hold. In this case the implants were coated with Proplast. The frozen jaws were chiseled free and Proplast-coated condyles were fastened with three screws on both sides of the jaw, forming artificial joints. The surgery was done by Dr. John N. Kent, associate professor of oral surgery at the University of Iowa, in Iowa City, Iowa and Dr. Edward C. Hinds, chairman of oral surgery, University of Texas, in Houston, Texas.

Dr. Kent believes that natural growth of bony tissue is now stabilizing the new joints. The patient can now open his mouth about an inch—"pretty good for an ankylosis patient," says Dr. Kent.

As a "side benefit" the young man no longer has a "bird chin" common to persons with frozen jaw problems. During the operation, his jaw was pulled forward into normal dental occlusion—"bite"—correcting the problem completely.

27. FACIAL SPASMS CONTROLLED WITH ACUPUNCTURE

WHEN CONVENTIONAL MEDICAL treatment proved unsuccessful in treating involuntary winking in one eye, ophthalmologist Dr. Joseph V. M. Ross, of Berwick, Pennsylvania, used acupuncture. He succeeded in four out of five cases where previously all other methods had failed.

The kind of winking under treatment was a muscular spasm of the face called medically, an *essential clonic facial spasm*. A spasm is called "essential" when no cause can be found.

Dr. Ross first gave thought to acupuncture several years ago when a Korean-born patient told him that years before, it had cured him of a persistent facial tick. Recalling that pressure points on the face are important in the treatment of this type of spasm, Dr. Ross reasoned that acupuncture might work if applied along the lines of those pressure points.

The success he had with his first patient encouraged him to extend the treatments. He has now treated five women patients between the ages of 38 and 64. Three of the patients were completely cured of the spasms. One has been free of them for two years, one for one year, and the other for five months. The fourth woman has not been completely cured, but her spasms are now less frequent and less severe.

The fifth patient, who also has had some mental problems in imagining illnesses (which couldn't be helped with psychiatric care), didn't get any help from the treatment.

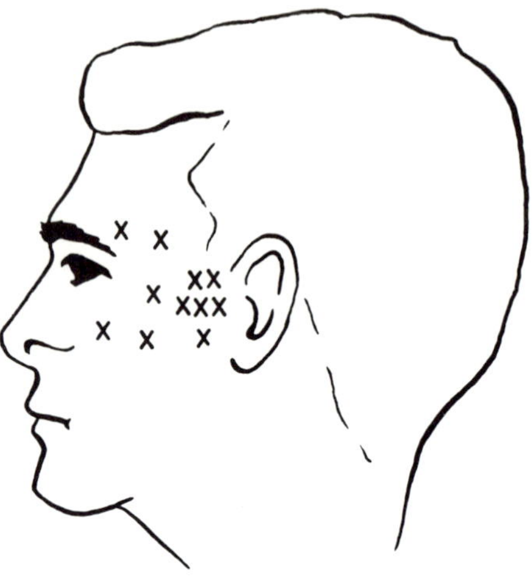

The acupuncture points drawn by Dr. Ross to outline his technique for controlling unilateral blepharospasm—one-side winking. The top set of needle points is used as a first alternative and the bottom set if the first do not produce the desired effect.

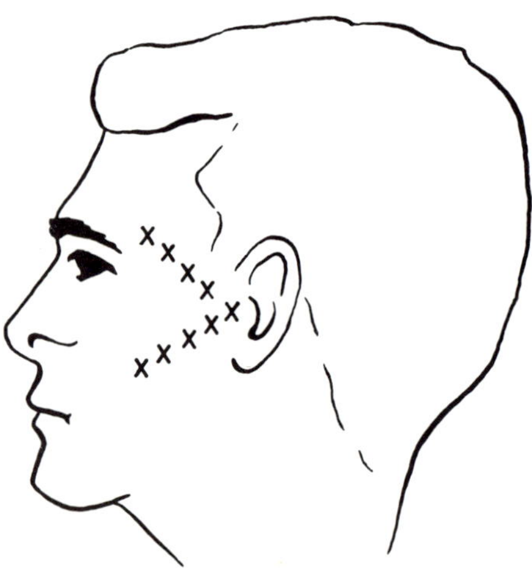

The acupuncture procedures were all executed by Dr. Ross in his office, and all patients were carefully briefed about the nature of the treatment and the fact that it was new and unproven.

For acupuncture needles, Dr. Ross used ordinary hypodermic needles, the kind normally used for injections. He inserted the needles in the spots he believed corresponded to the pressure points, and left them in for 10 minutes (Dr. Ross does not twirl the needles as is said to be done by the Chinese physicians.) In general, the needles were inserted to a depth of ¼ to ½ inches.

After the needles are in place, Dr. Ross insists that the patient look at himself in a mirror. Since the causes of this facial tick are not known, Dr. Ross reasons that if there is any psychological reason for the spasm there might be some psychological value for the patient to see himself in the mirror when the needles are all in place.

At the end of the treatment, the needles are simply removed—no bandages are necessary. The patients are instructed to wash treated areas with soap, water and rubbing alcohol four times daily for several days.

Dr. Ross says that he has no explanations for "the mechanism of action of acupuncture." He doubts if the acupuncture treatment would be effective in cases of bilateral spasms (on both sides of the face), although he has not tried it. He has several patients who suffer from the bilateral spasms, but none were willing to volunteer for the acupuncture treatment.

28. SUCCESS WITH FROZEN SPERM FROM SEMEN BANKS

MANY MEN ARE NOT AWARE that certain medical procedures may affect their future fertility. These procedures involve surgery, radiation therapy, chemotherapy, or a combination of these. Such surgical procedures as bladder neck surgery and prostatectomy may cause loss of semen as it goes into the bladder instead of the urethra, following the operations. Operations on a cancer of the testicles may cause sterility, without impairing the capacity for erection and orgasm. Radiation to the region of the testicles may cause permanent genetic damage and chemotherapy for leukemia and Hodgkins disease may have a lasting effect on the quality of semen. There are many other procedures which may cause a loss of fertility, or impair the quality of semen.

Doctors don't talk to patients about this possible loss of fertility, because they do not think anything can be done about the situation. Recently, however, many doctors have become aware that it is now possible to preserve human sperm (semen) by freezing it, and then using it at some later date to cause conception.

The use of frozen human sperm to create a pregnancy is not very new, but many doctors are not aware of its successful use because only some 500 babies have resulted from artificial insemination with frozen sperm over the past twenty years.

Recently conducted studies of artificial insemination with

frozen, human sperm have proved that there is no danger of birth defects in the children born as its result. The number— and kind—of birth defects in children born out of use of frozen human sperm is the same as in children born from ordinary pregnancy. The latest figures on this important question have come from Dr. Samuel J. Behrman, director of the Center for Research in Reproductive Biology at the University of Michigan in Ann Arbor.

Dr. Behrman recently concluded a study during which he supervised 104 pregnancies which resulted from artificial inseminations with frozen human sperm. The mothers produced 98 healthy babies, including one set of twins. Two of the babies were born with birth defects, and of those, one was a hereditary condition which the mother had, and the other had an imperforate hymen, which is not considered a serious birth defect. The other six pregnancies terminated with miscarriages during the first six to eight weeks—a miscarriage rate which is only half of that normally expected.

Dr. Behrman's overall study involved 200 women. Therefore, these 104 pregnancies represent a successful impregnation rate of 52%. While this rate of success is lower than the rate of success achieved with freshly donated semen, it definitely proves that frozen human sperm is effective.

The question of how long human semen can remain fertile while frozen has no definite answer at the moment. The methods of freezing it and thawing it out are important to preserving the fertility of stored semen. Studies—proven by conception—have shown that it has remained fertile for as long as 10 years.

In the opinion of Dr. Jerome A. Silbert, director of laboratories of the IDANT Corp., a New York City sperm bank, storage at dry ice temperature can keep the sperm fertile only slightly longer than one year. However, using liquid nitrogen (which creates twice the cold of dry ice) for storage, fertility can be preserved for years.

Storing frozen semen for possible future use—a sort of "infertility insurance"—may one day become a common procedure. Already there are semen banks in New York, Los Angeles, Chicago, San Francisco, Minneapolis, Ann Arbor, Dallas and a number of other cities.

29. OVERCOMING FEAR OF FLIGHT

FEAR OF FLYING is a common malady in the jet age. Many persons have an instinctive fear of flying which is so deep that it is almost impossible for them to get on an airplane, even if they strongly desire to do so.

Fear of flying affects different people to different degrees, and many travelers apply home remedies, such as double shots of whiskey, taken at regular intervals before boarding.

In flight, they imbibe of generous quantities by way of sedative. Alcohol gives temporary relief to some people, but, unfortunately, the fear of flying is so deeply ingrained in some of them that the alcohol treatment is of no help.

Psychiatrists have been unable to agree on the causes of fear of flying, but it is apparently an involuntary fear. Most persons afflicted with this fear can't trace the fear to any specific incident. Most sufferers become anxious or terrified at different phases of the flight. Some react as soon as the plane's door is shut; others are terrified at the take-off; and many panic at the grinding sound of the landing gear being raised. Turbulence scares many people; others break out in a sweat watching the runway during landing.

Various psychiatrists have tried different methods of relieving this fear. Dr. Monte J. Meldman of Forest Hospital in Des Plaines, Illinois, has found the use of an analgesic (pain-relieving drug) coupled with flying imagery successful in controlling a person's fear of flying.

The patient is given penthrane, an analgesic drug in gas form, through a vaporizer and mask placed over his face. After breathing in the gas for one minute the patient gets a mild feeling of intoxication and giddiness.

Prior to the inhalation of the gas, the patient has an interview with Dr. Meldman. He tells the doctor his memories about flying, describing different feelings of fear or anxiety that were connected with different flying experiences. The doctor makes a list of these memories, and after the gas starts to work, he asks the person under treatment to recall those memories.

The memories are recalled one after the other, starting with the most severe. As each memory is recalled, the patient takes two or three deep inhalations of the penthrane gas. Each session includes five selected memories which are quenched by whiffs of the gas.

After the "memory quenching" the patient is instructed to imagine pleasant flying experiences. This imagery includes packing for the trip, travelling to the airport, take-off, and completion of the flight. Specific instructions are given to the patient for relaxation and enjoyment during the imagined flying experience.

According to Dr. Meldman, regular inhalation of penthrane gas produces deep muscular relaxation. "This experience of relaxation," he says, "is associated with a pleasurable feeling, and patients respond to it favorably, very often feeling somewhat giddy and high."

Dr. Meldman tells of the case of a 37-year-old woman whose fear of flying became a great problem because her parents lived in California and she lived in Chicago. She had to make frequent trips to California due to the parents' illness.

"She had chickened-out of visiting them the summer before she entered treatment," Dr. Meldman said, "and this was a bitter blow to her, because she was supposed to go home but was so terrified that she couldn't go to the airport and get on the plane.

"Before that episode," he continued, "she had flown infrequently, but suffered a great deal of anxiety before each flight. She said she did not mind the time spent in the air as much as the anticipation period before going out to the airport. This feeling of anxiety and uneasiness lasted from the time she knew she would take a flight until the flight was over —as much as two weeks."

Dr. Meldman treated this patient by having her remember her unpleasant experiences while inhaling penthrane gas. The gas was also administered while the woman imagined future pleasant experiences with flying.

After receiving 16 one-half hour treatments the woman took a flight to Florida with little difficulty. She subsequently took flights to Michigan and California. She sent a letter to Dr. Meldman telling him she had experienced normal excitement for her trip and has been able to fly since then without difficulty.

30. A READING AND WRITING SYSTEM FOR THE BLIND

PERSONS WHO HAVE no light perception at all are totally blind as well as legally blind, but those who have some light perception can manage a limited level of reading capability even if they have only 5% to 10% left of their visual sense still active. They can often read either specially prepared material in large type, or even smaller print (8 to 10 point type) if it is held about ½" from their eyes.

However, even for those who can manage this limited level of reading capability, there are many frustrations and difficulties. Sometimes, inadequate illumination reaches the printed surface because it is blocked by the reader's head. Often, writing is difficult because one can't see what he is writing. These types of difficulties lead to fatigue and frustration.

A new device, called the Visualtek Read/Write System, permits many persons legally blind—but who have some light perception—to read newspapers, books, and magazines as well as to take notes. They are even able to use a typewriter. The new creation allows persons with even severe visual impairments (even those with as little as ½ or 1 percent residual vision) to live somewhat normally.

The unit consists of a movable viewing table and a TV

Additional material touching on this subject can be found in chapters 9, 21, 25, 36, 56 and 70.

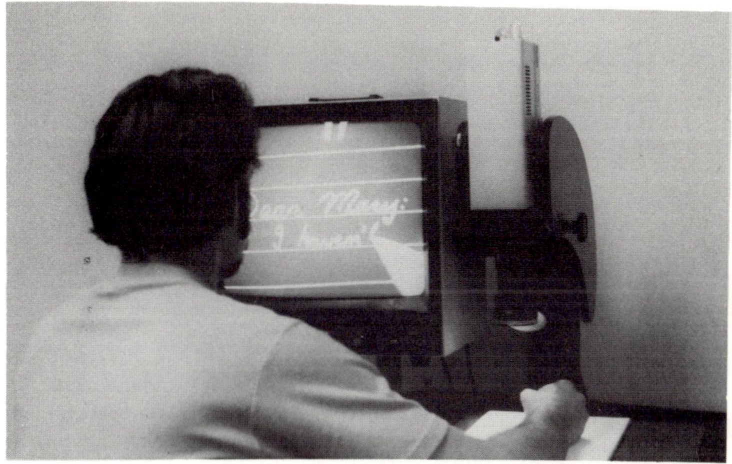

A Visualtek Read/Write System used to handwrite a letter. The user keeps his eye on the screen, not the letter.

monitor. (It can also be used with an ordinary TV set.) It magnifies up to 45 times and sharpens the clarity of virtually any material. Letters can be enlarged by the user up to 3" high, and still maintain a sharp contrast between the letters and the background. The machine is a compact portable which can be placed on a desk or tabletop, taken to the classroom or to the library.

To use the device, the operator puts the material he wants to read on the viewing table. A closed circuit TV camera "scans" the material and projects an enlarged image of it on the TV-like screen of the monitor. Virtually anything to be read (or written on) is placed under the equipment: books, magazines, newspapers, forms to be filled out . . . even the label on a pill bottle.

The magnification is easily adjusted. The viewing table is moved from side to side and front to back, allowing the reader to scan an entire page without touching the material.

Writing is accomplished by placing a writing pad on the viewing table and the written material can be followed by looking at the monitor screen.

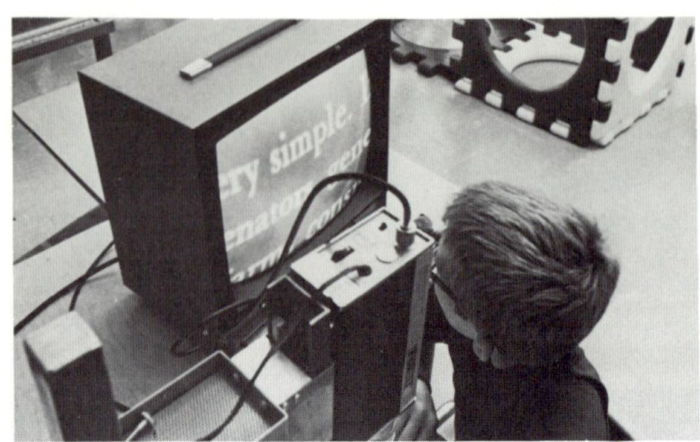

A 12-year-old using the Visualtek System to read a book printed in regular type.

An accessory is available which allows the device to be used with a typewriter. The individual can see what he is typing while it's being typed, and he can quickly proofread and make corrections as required.

The equipment is also capable of reversing the image. If the ordinary printed page were magnified, the screen would be almost entirely light (corresponding to the background color of the paper), with dark areas corresponding to the information being read. Typically, 80-90% of the screen would be light, and this constitutes an extremely annoying glare to the person with limited vision. In some cases, prolonged viewing of such a screen at close distances can cause nausea or excessive fatigue.

The answer to this problem is to provide reversed, or negative, images. Electronically, white and black areas are interchanged, so that the background (and therefore 80-90% of the display screen) is dark, while only the letters of the words being read are displayed in high contrast white. Such image reversal is essential for those with severely limited vision.

Price of the unit ranges from $900 to $1,500, depending upon accessories. The system is available from Visualtek, 1901 Olympic Blvd., Santa Monica, California 90404.

31. RETRAINING PARALYZED MUSCLES AT HOME

THE USE OF *electromyography* to re-educate paralyzed muscles is more than ten years old, but lack of simple, inexpensive equipment has limited its application. Another obstacle is the lack of trained therapists in *neuromuscular facilitation*—the use of reflexes to achieve movement.

The principle of electromyography is simple: A human muscle produces electric current when it contracts. Even if only a few fibres in the muscle contract—a motion so gentle that it isn't even felt by the person doing it—there will be some current generated by that gentle contraction.

The current which is generated by the muscles is picked up by electrodes which are either needles inserted into the muscle, or metal plates pasted on the surface of the skin. The current picked up by the electrodes is sent to the amplifier, to the converter, and out through a loudspeaker. In this manner a person can hear his muscles if they are working at all—no matter how feebly.

Muscles contract when a coded "message" travels from the brain to the muscle. These messages travel from the brain down the spinal cord to the muscle, and these messages are present in many patients even though they are not able to contract specific muscles.

Additional material touching on this subject can be found in chapter 97.

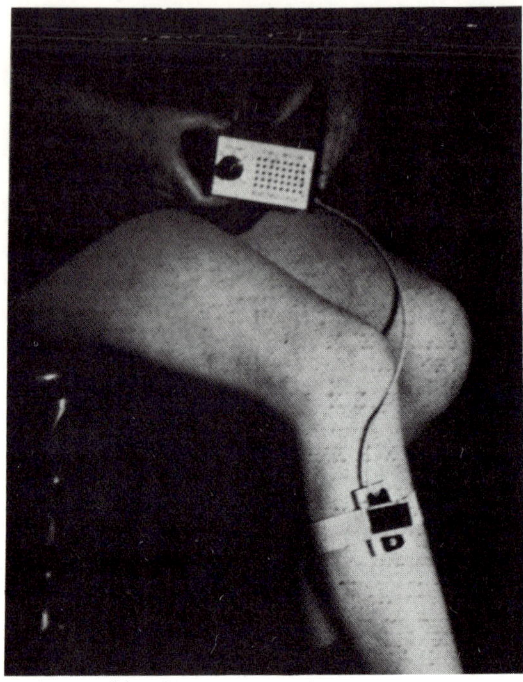

A portable electromyography monitor in use.

Electromyography machines convert these messages into sound so that the patient can hear when the messages are being sent from the brain. When the patient with a paralyzed muscle hears the sound, he concentrates on making that sound again, and these continued efforts to make that same sound are eventually transferred into movement. In this way, the patient may be able to re-learn to use his muscles.

Learning to use this sound (which is a converted reflex) to produce movement requires expert assistance from a physician and from a therapist trained in neuromuscular facilitation. However, not all exercise sessions require this assistance, and if a patient were able to do some of them at home he would have more time for other therapy which is needed to round out the training program.

This home training is now possible with a simple, inexpensive portable *electromyographic monitor* devised by an engineer, Larry Frazier, for the Casa Colina Hospital for Rehabilitative Medicine in Pomona, Calif. The unit is compact, easy to operate—and costs around $250. It is battery-operated, and consists of a loud-speaker, volume control, and a sensor unit with an electrode.

The sensor unit, equipped with an electrode plate on one side, is taped or strapped over the area to be monitored and then plugged into the volume control box. This has a "volume" control which can be increased until the sound is heard. The patient then concentrates on increasing the number and volume of the popping sounds.

According to Dr. Herbert F. Johnson, clinical director of the hospital, the equipment has produced encouraging results. In all but one of the patients who used the equipment in the initial trials, there was a return of "significant function" in a previously paralyzed muscle.

The monitor is now on the market and available from Electro Labs of Pomona, Calif.

32. PACEMAKERS
FOR THE ELDERLY

OLDER PERSONS often continue to suffer from heart disease for which younger persons have been able to get relief by having electronic pacemakers implanted in their chests. Doctors have feared that the old or infirm would be unable to survive the surgery necessary for implantation of the pacemaker.

Now Dr. Gerald C. Timmis, of William Beaumont Hospital in Royal Oak, Michigan, reports that elderly patients are "prime candidates" for permanent heart pacemakers.

A new technique of implantation is responsible for the change in attitude. Earlier, implantation required surgery. The wall of the chest had to be cut open so that the wires of the pacemaker could be properly attached to the heart. Older people, already weakened by heart disease, were, at best, not good candidates for pacemakers.

A new technique, first developed about six years ago, is called *transvenous endocardial pacing*, and it does not require major surgery. (*Transvenous* means through the vein; *endocardial* means inside the heart.) A small slit is made in the skin of the chest to form a "pocket" for the pacemaker. This simple procedure is performed while the patient is under local anesthesia. The electrode—the wire from the pacemaker to

Additional material touching on this subject can be found in chapters 7, 24, 46, 84, 94, 96, 98 and 99.

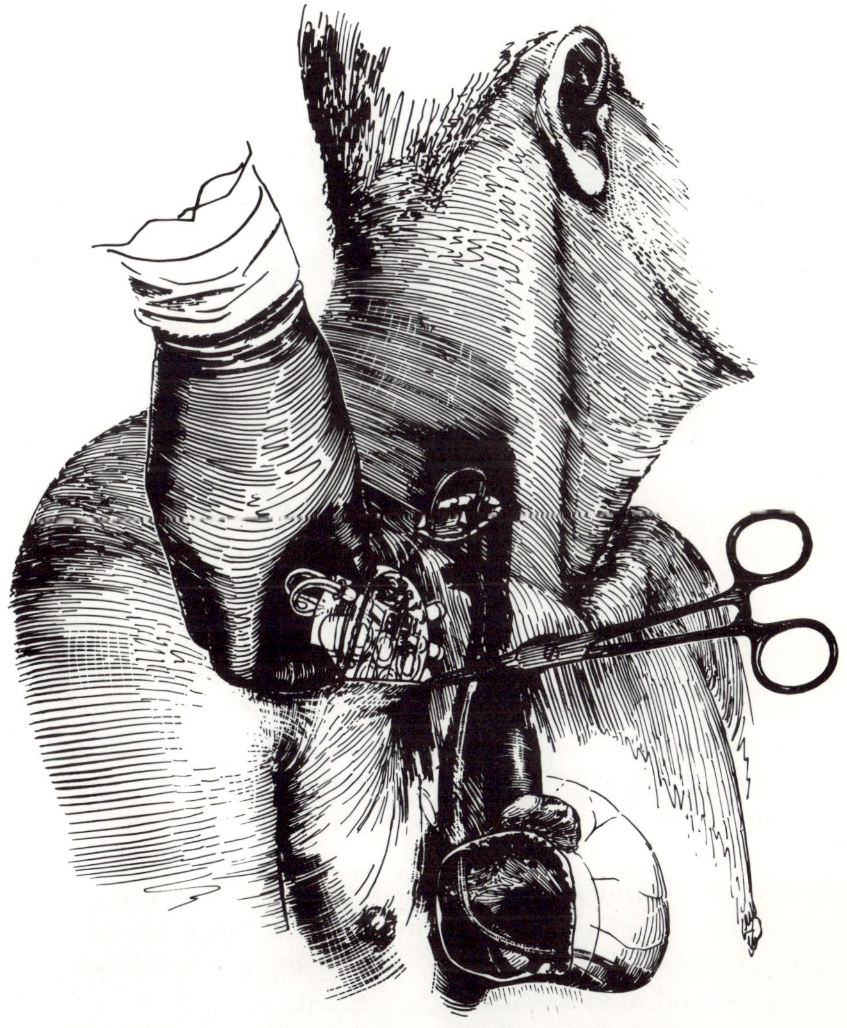

The implantation of a transvenous pacemaker. The pacemaker is placed in a skin "pocket" in the chest. The ends of the wire—the electrode—can be seen inside the heart, in the right ventricle.

the heart—is slipped into the heart by guiding it in through a vein in the neck.

To insert the wire into the vein, a hollow, needle-like tube

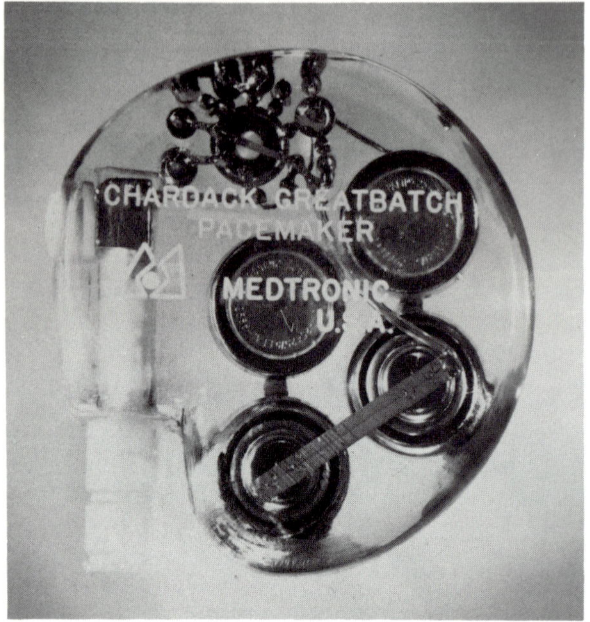

An implantable pacemaker.

is inserted into the vein, and the wire—which is very fine—is inserted into the vein through the tube. There is no need to cut the vein. When the wire reaches the inside of the heart, it is manipulated by the surgeon until it is in the proper position.

Doctor Timmis has installed pacemakers, using this technique, in about 80 patients whose average age was 73 years. All suffered from various degrees of heart blockage, often complicated by Stokes-Adams attacks and other heart diseases. Sixty-eight of these patients were subjects of a follow-up study by Dr. Timmis.

Sixty-three of them recovered sufficiently to be discharged from the hospital, and 57 had "significantly improved." Doctor Timmis says that he is "impressed with the generally gratifying results with this wonderful group of people."

33. A REVOLUTIONARY PLASTIC SPIRAL BRACE

FOR THE FIRST TIME in over a hundred years, the design of leg braces is undergoing a revolutionary change. The reason for these new designs lies in recent studies of human locomotion—the manner in which people walk.

These studies disclosed that when people walk, their legs are subject to a rotating motion. As they step forward, the leg not only moves forward but actually rotates along its axis. This is called *transverse rotation*—the same sort of motion that is produced by the winding and unwinding of a spiral.

Because there is often a considerable amount of transverse rotation between the hip and the foot, authorities feel that it should be taken into consideration in designing braces. However, most conventional braces still restrict motion to one direction.

A new plastic spiral brace, designed by New York University's Institute of Rehabilitation Medicine, provides for the control of transverse rotation. The brace, suitable for the lower leg, and medically called a *below-knee orthosis* is made of tough, flexible plastic and is spiral-shaped. The design allows it to wind and unwind, following the natural transverse rotation of the leg.

The brace is made of one piece of an acrylic-nylon material with a horizontal band attached to the spiral at the level of the

---

Additional material touching on this subject can be found in chapter 19.

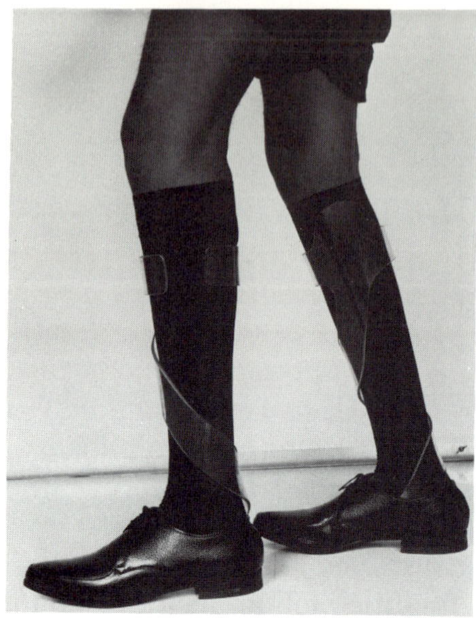

The plastic spiral brace in use.

calf. The base of the brace is a foot-like piece which provides normal, built-in foot support, and it can be worn with all types of shoes. Since it is a unit in itself, it can be used with a variety of shoes, and not just one type. The brace weighs only six and one-half ounces.

The brace's advantage as an improved walking aid is very important, but two other important factors are its appeareance and the psychological effect it has for its users. Suddenly, rid of the unsightly steel bars of which metal braces are normally built, the users no longer think or feel that they are cripples. Many users also report that the spiral is very comfortable and its light weight very pleasant and easy to handle.

The new plastic brace is ideal for persons who lack motor control in the ankle—except in severe spasticity. However, the brace can also be used in conditions involving weakness of only one group of muscles, rather than total paralysis.

34. A "STIMULATOR" TO CONTROL PAIN

THE USE BY Governor Wallace, of Alabama, of a "stimulator" to control pain, and his reported satisfaction with it, has called public attention to a machine used by Dr. Ross Davis, Chief of the Spinal Cord Injury Service at the Veterans Administration Hospital in Miami, Florida.

Called a *cutaneous* (skin) *stimulator*, the small, battery-operated device does just what its name implies: It stimulates the skin by producing a mild, tingling sensation. This tingling, if the stimulator is adjusted properly, is not unpleasant, and some patients have even described it as being pleasant.

The device is a small box—about the size of a transistor radio—containing two size D, flashlight batteries and a pulse generator which converts the low battery voltage to higher voltage pulsations. These reach the skin via electrodes attached by leads to the box. Two dial controls on the box allow the patient to control the strength and frequency of the impulses to counteract the pain.

The electrodes are taped onto the skin. An electrolyte solution is applied between the electrodes and the skin to insure good contact. With some patients, it is necessary to stimulate larger areas of skin than can now be done wih the standard electrodes that come with the present-day devices that are

---

Additional material touching on this subject can be found in chapters 57 and 85.

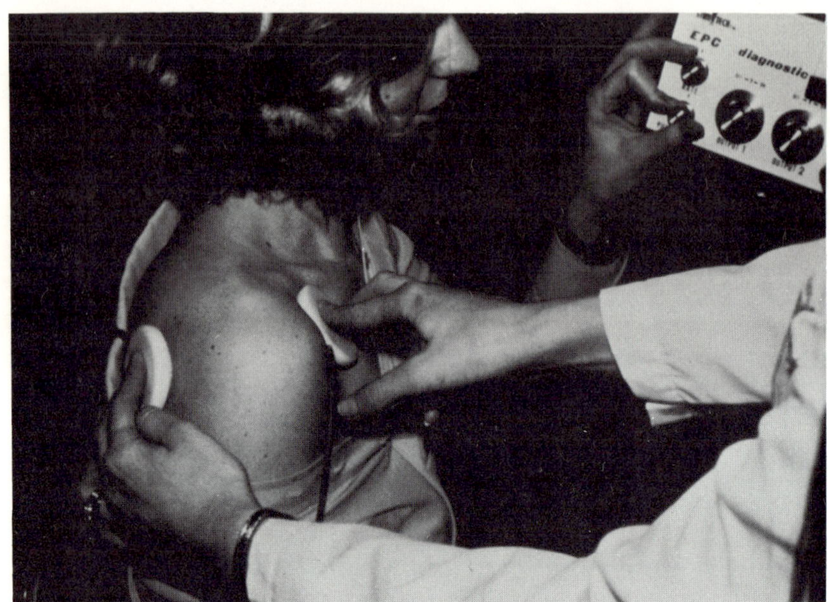

Modified length electrode strips taped to the back of a paraplegic patient suffering from backpain in the area marked. A Medtronics Cutaneous Stimulator is shown in the lower right hand corner.

commercially available. For these patients, Dr. Davis has developed special electrodes, about 11 inches long, one to two inches wide, and 7/16" thick. These are made of foam padding impregnated with electrolyte cream and backed with aluminum foil. The special electrodes are custom-made at the VA hospital.

In use, the electrodes are placed over the general pain area —some "trial-and-error" placements are needed to locate the spot where they give the most relief. The electrodes can be left in place all day, and even at night, but a different spot on the skin has to be used each day as the paste can cause a slight skin reaction if the electrode is pasted in the same spot a couple of days in a row. Once the electrodes are in place, the patient switches on the stimulator.

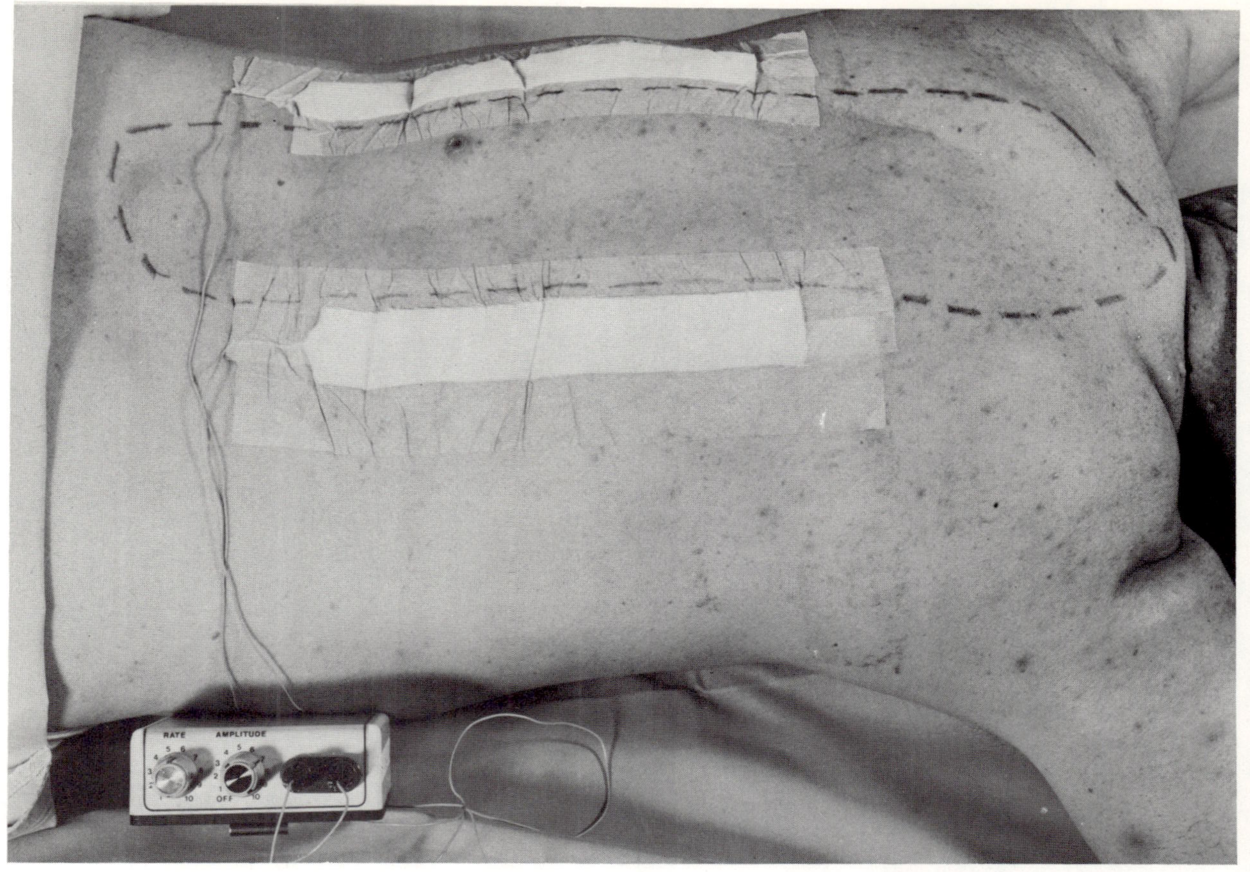

A Stimtech Personal Stimulator. This one costs around $250.00.

There is no question that the stimulator does help some persons. Governor Wallace reported pain relief, and Dr. Davis reports the chances of the device helping the governor were about two to one. Dr. Davis also reported that, of the spinal cord injury patients whom he equipped with the device, approximately half have had definite pain relief—enough relief so that they didn't have to take any more pain-killing drugs. Another 10% to 20% have had *some* pain relief. These relief figures, however, are a verbal report—no figures have yet been published in any medical journal.

How, and why, the stimulator works is uncertain. Possibly, the tingling stimulates the nerves in the skin to cancel out the pain impulses. Or, the tingling sensation may take precedence over pain.

Besides treating patients with spinal cord injuries, Dr. Davis has also used the stimulator to treat frozen shoulder cases, persons who had pain after multiple lumbar disc surgery, and patients with nerve damage in various parts of the body.

The stimulator is now being commercially marketed by several companies whose names and addresses may be obtained from the Miami VA hospital. Readers interested in this device are advised to first consult with their doctors.

35. RAPID RECOVERY CATARACT SURGERY

A NEW METHOD of cataract surgery has been developed by Dr. Charles Kelman of the Manhattan Eye, Ear, Nose and Throat Hospital in New York City.

The new technique permits the patient to return to normal activity the day after surgery, while conventional surgery requires a week in the hospital and several weeks of convalescence at home. The new procedure is as safe as conventional surgery.

Dr. Kelman invented the procedure and the equipment used in the operation. It is basically a complex computerized machine equipped with a hand-held ultrasonic probe. The probe is the instrument used in the surgery.

The probe is inserted into the eye through a single, tiny incision. In the probe is a hollow needle that vibrates 40,000 times per second. Each tap of the needle's tip dissolves a microscopic fragment of the cataract and then sucks up the liquid as if through a straw.

The actual operation is very quick. With young patients, the withdrawal takes about a minute. Older patients, with hardened cataracts, require up to five minutes.

The machine automatically controls most functions of the probe. The strength of the suction, for example, is automatically controlled so that if the tip of the needle hits a

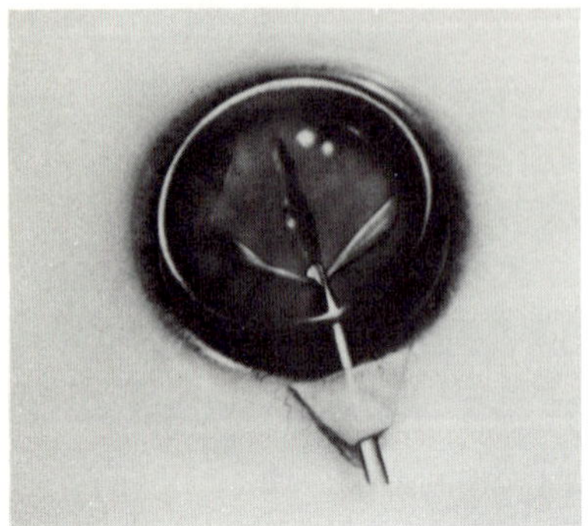

A cystotome withdraws a V-shaped piece of anterior capsule.

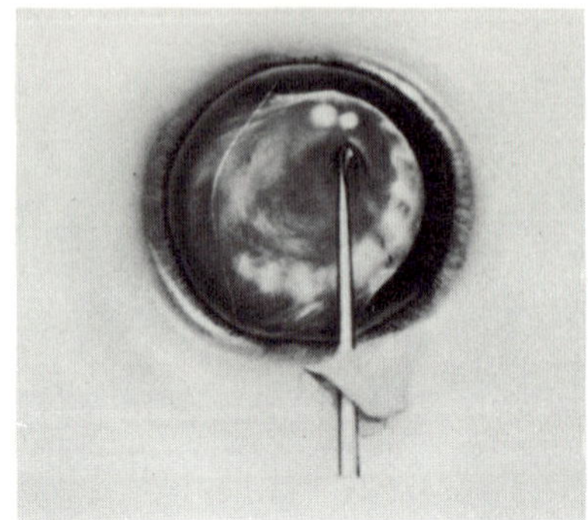

An irrigating hook prolapses the nucleus into the anterior chamber.

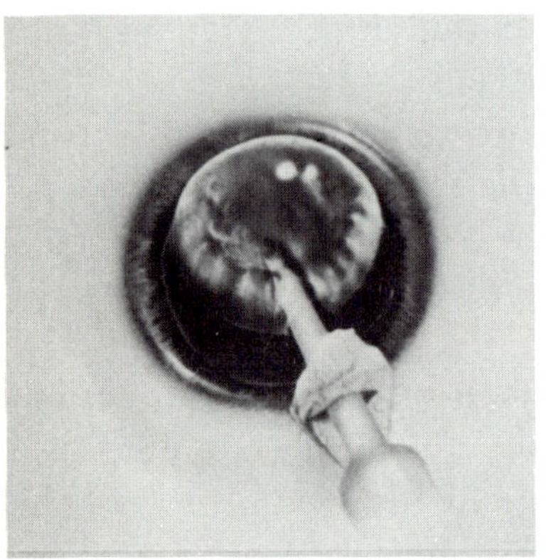

The titanium tip of the handpiece is placed behind the nucleus to emulsify and aspirate the lens.

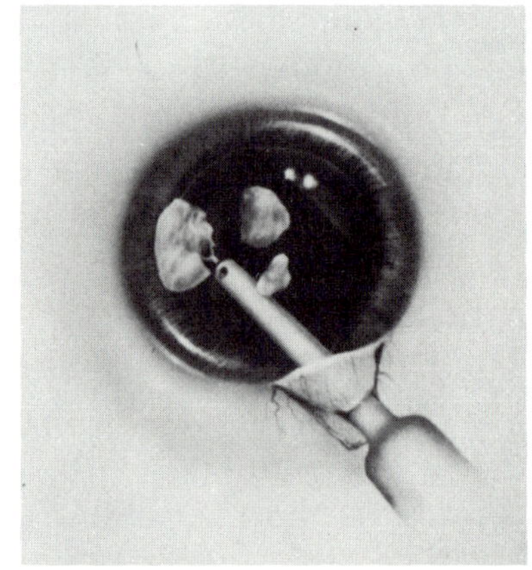

The lens fragments.

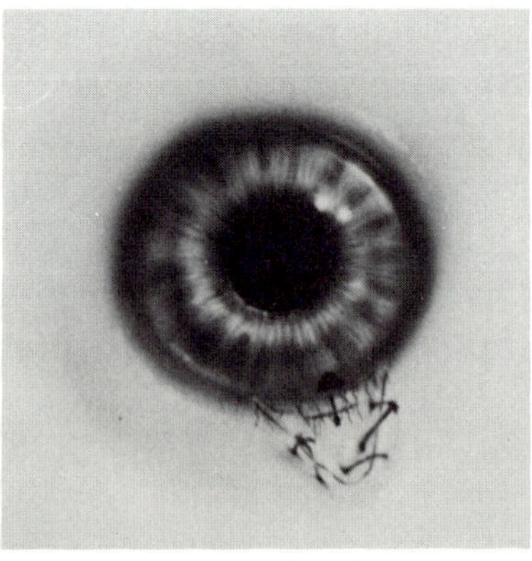

The incision is closed with one suture.

harder piece of the cataract, the suction power is increased to help suck it out more easily.

The machine costs about $40,000 and 34 are currently in use throughout this country and in England.

The new technique, which is done under a microscope, requires a very steady hand in order to pass the drill through the very tiny cut in the eye which is generally about 1/16 to 1/8 of an inch. Surgeons, who want to use the machines, are taught the technique by Dr. Kelman himself.

Some 200 surgeons have already been trained in the new procedure and have performed more than 4,000 operations throughout the country. Dr. Kelman himself has performed over 800 of them.

36. ULTRASONIC OBSTACLE DETECTOR FOR THE BLIND

A BLIND CANADIAN scientist has invented a small, hand-held, obstacle detector for the blind.

James Swail, 25-year veteran of the staff of the National Research Council of Canada in Ottawa, has engineered a number of instruments which aid the blind. His most recent is the *ultrasonic obstacle detector*.

The detector is Jim Swail's approach to the blind man's problem of how to move about in populated areas without the traditional long, white cane or the seeing-eye dog. There are certain situations where both the cane and the dog become, in Jim's words, "socially unacceptable."

Indoors, in a crowded house party setting, for example, the cane tends to trip people, and it becomes a bit of a nuisance to have around. The same applies to the dog.

A similar situation occurs when a blind man tries to navigate between rows of tables in a restaurant. He lives with the fear that his cane, in searching out obstacles, will inadvertently slide under one of the tables and touch another person. Such occasions become terribly embarrassing.

In such situations, but more generally, when a blind person is *not* called upon to move quickly nor perform actions calling for much care and attention (i.e., scanning an office or cor-

---

Additional material touching on this subject can be found in chapters 9, 21, 25, 56 and 70.

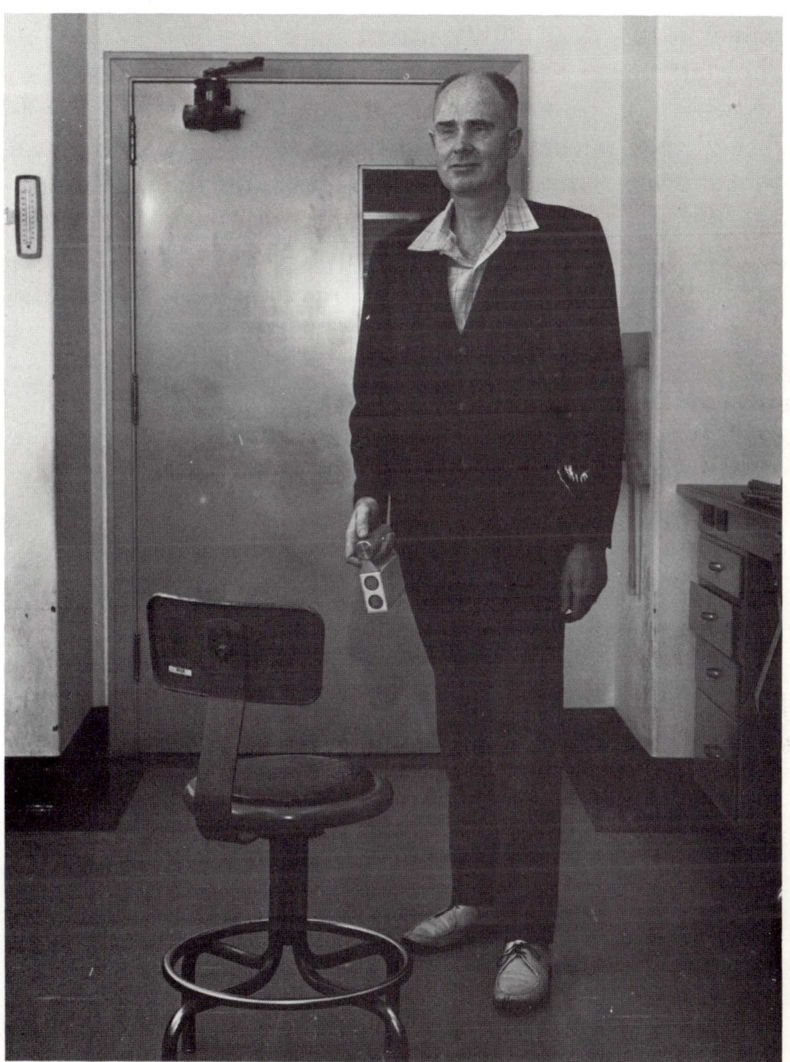

A patient demonstrating the ultrasonic obstacle detector.

ridor for newly-placed or disarranged articles such as chairs, tables, wastebaskets, etc.), the hand-held ultrasonic detector is expected to prove highly useful.

The detector is essentially a simple radar unit similar to those used for remote television channel switching. It is packaged in a pocket-sized plastic carrying case, and has a handle. Power comes from built-in, rechargeable batteries.

The device sends out a narrow, invisible beam of sound, which bounces off objects and returns to the detector. This action causes a rod to vibrate through a hole in the unit's handle and against the forefinger of the operator.

The distance to a target is estimated by altering the range control until the vibration stops. The ranges are set at four, seven and 15 feet, and the receiver unit will respond to targets within the selected range. Target (object) direction is determined by scanning.

37. MORE MOBILITY
   FOR THE HANDICAPPED

FOR THE HANDICAPPED, confined to a wheelchair, the wheelchair often becomes a prison. The handicapped person is almost immobile in a world that lives on mobility—walking, riding or flying. Of course, many handicapped persons can drive a car. In the past, they have needed the help of others to get in and out; not any more, however.

A Fort Lauderdale, Florida firm, the only one of its kind in the United States, is converting Chevrolet or GMC sliding door vans to vehicles that give new independence and freedom to those confined to wheelchairs.

Now, such a person can wheel his chair to the van, and by operating outside controls at the rear of the vehicle, can open the doors and then, with the flick of a switch, operate a lift large enough to hold a wheelchair. The lift descends automatically. The user then covers and locks the outside control box, and drives the wheelchair onto the lift. Controls on the lift bring the wheelchair and its passenger up to the level of the van's floorbed, and swing the lift inside the van. (The wheelchair is automatically locked into the lift while being swung up and in.)

Once inside the van, the driver directs his wheelchair toward the position ordinarily occupied by the driver's seat—which has been removed. In this position, the driver flips

---

Additional material touching on this subject can be found in chapters 8 and 66.

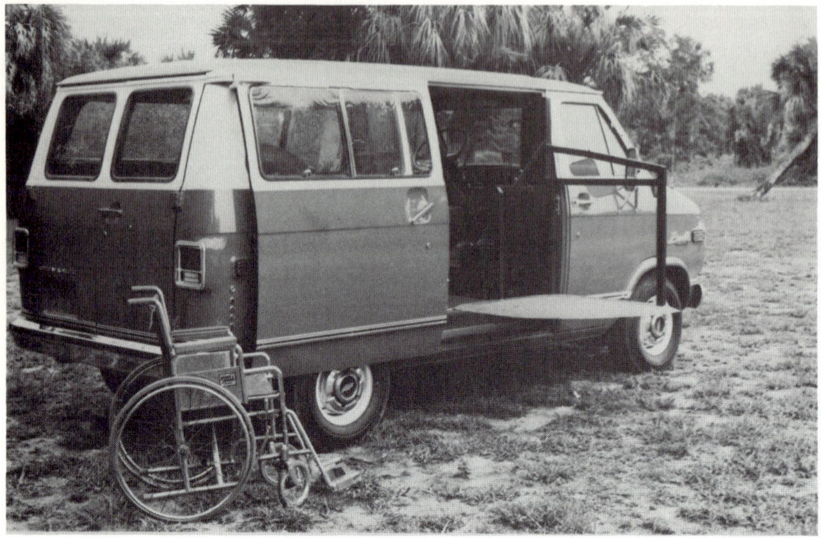

A Chevrolet van equipped with a wheel chair lifting device. The driving seat can be modified according to the incapacity of the driver.

switches which close and lock the door. (By use of controls inside, another descent of the lift can be made for other passengers.)

When the driver pulls his chair into the space ordinarily occupied by the driver's seat, it is engaged by clamps that automatically lock it into correct driving position. Shifting and other controls are console mounted in a position easily accessible to the driver. Various steering and other accessories are available, tailored to the individual driver's wishes and his disability.

Does the converted van work? The proof is in the fact that the firm's sales manager, a quadriplegic, regularly drives such a converted van while going about his business.

The conversions are available in various styles, including a drop-floor model for persons who are too tall for the regular van.

A lift-only conversion (where the handicapped is only a

passenger) is a simple project and is available in a kit package requiring about four hours to install. However, if the handicapped is interested in driving himself, a full conversion is needed, and that is best done locally, at Fort Lauderdale.

Full conversion only takes about a week, and various arrangements can be made such as, for example, pricing the van locally and sending the specifications to Fort Lauderdale, where an identical vehicle can be furnished at the same price. The cost of conversion varies according to individual needs, but a standard full conversion runs about $1,800. Interested readers may write for information to Helper Industries, Inc., 832 N.W. 1st Street, Ft. Lauderdale, Florida.

38. CRYOSURGERY MAY PREVENT CANCER OF THE CERVIX

CRYOSURGERY has a new use: treatment of localized cancer of the cervix.

Cryosurgery is the use of cold as a knife (*cryo* means cold). It is performed with a cryoprobe—an ice knife—a metal spear that looks like a crochet needle. It is a long needle, heavily insulated, and only the tip is uncovered. The needle is hollow inside—it's really a thin tube with a bare, sharply pointed tip. The probe is connected to a machine—or container—that produces the cold for the tip of the needle.

The cold is produced by liquid gasses—nitrogen or freon—either packed into a container or produced on the spot by a machine. This depends on the gas and the degree of cold required for a particular job.

To operate, the liquid nitrogen is pumped into the cryoprobe all the way up to the open tip. The tip becomes so cold that it can freeze any part of the body it touches. The surgeon either touches the tip of the cryoprobe to the part he wants to cut out, or he sprays that part with the liquid nitrogen. In either case, this freezes the tissue. The frozen tissue can then be scraped off or it sloughs off by itself. There is no bleeding in cryosurgery; it is painless and requires no anesthesia.

Additional material touching on this subject can be found in chapters 14, 15, 16, 65 and 93.

Dr. William C. Crisp of the University of Arizona-Maricopa County General Hospital in Phoenix, Arizona says there are many advantages to cryosurgery:

"Cryosurgery is safe and easy to use in a wide variety of lesions, both cancerous and benign (non-cancerous). Because nerve ends are destroyed quickly in cryosurgery, it is relatively painless and there is very little bleeding. Also, cryosurgery is inexpensive and the majority of the patients can be treated in the hospital's outpatient department with no anesthesia."

Only localized cervical cancer, medically called *carcinoma in situ*, can be treated by cryosurgery. Cancer of the cervix which is spread out into the uterus, called *invasive cancer*, cannot be treated with this technique.

In the actual operation, the *cryoprobe* is used to spray the cancer tumor with liquid nitrogen for a very short period of time. The intense cold of the liquid nitrogen—its temperature can be brought down to *minus* 320°F—kills the cancer. The entire procedure takes less than half an hour.

Doctor Crisp uses cryosurgery for treatment of localized cervical cancer and in the treatment of dysplasia (abnormal tissue growth). A follow-up study of 193 patients—151 with dysplasia and 42 with carcinoma in situ—made by Dr. Crisp, yielded very good results. "After six years," said Dr. Crisp, "I have seen no recurrence to the conditions in over 94% of my patients."

Dr. Crisp believes that cryosurgery is the ideal cancer-preventive treatment for the younger woman who wants to have children, but is suffering from conditions of the cervix known as *congenital erosion* or *postpartum erosion*. Congenital erosion happens after the start of menstruation, while postpartum erosion occurs immediately after giving birth for the first time. Both conditions involve growth of sensitive tissue which is known to be particularly susceptible to cancer.

According to Dr. Crisp, this sensitive tissue can be destroyed with cryosurgery, causing the body to replace it with a stronger tissue, no longer cancer-prone. This can be done without reducing the fertility or endangering normal functions of the uterus, while at the same time reducing the probability of cervical cancer in the future.

Cryosurgery can also be used to treat terminal cancer cases. In terminal cancer of the cervix—where no hope exists for the patient of any cure—cryosurgery reduces the size of the tumor, controlling discharge and bleeding and decreasing pain. These terminal cancer tumors can be frozen with cryosurgery and refrozen after they have again grown larger without serious problems.

39. CHILDREN WITH LEUKEMIA

ALL—A TYPE OF BLOOD cancer more technically known as *acute lymphotic leukemia*—is the most common childhood cancer. Each year it kills some 2,000 children in this country. Twenty-five years ago, children with ALL survived only a few weeks or months.

In the late 1940s a new method to fight ALL was first introduced; *chemotherapy*—the use of combinations of chemicals and drugs in treatment. As the new technique continued to improve, the life expectancy of ALL-afflicted children became extended. Now, the new method has been developed to a point where 50 per cent of the children with ALL should survive for at least five years, and a number of them might even be cured—if they get the specialized treatment now required. Unfortunately, only about fifteen per cent of the children afflicted with ALL get the best treatment known today. The specialized treatment is difficult and expensive, and only about 40 institutions in the country have experience with the new procedures. The powerful drugs used in chemotherapy are dangerous if improperly used, and many tests and observations are continuously required when a child is undergoing treatment. The best place to treat the child is in one of the specialized research centers.

Additional material touching on this subject can be found in chapter 45.

In the case of ALL, "being a guinea pig" is very much an advantage, according to Dr. James F. Holland, chairman of an international group of researchers and Chairman of the Department of Neoplastic Diseases at the Mount Sinai School of Medicine in New York. "The children need have no fear of being in new and experimental treatments since they do much better than the others," says Dr. Holland.

Though it is impossible for all children with ALL to attend the specialized centers, many of the centers will start the treatment and then it can be continued by the child's personal doctor who can keep in touch with the center for advice and instructions. It is not even necessary to be admitted to a hospital to be treated at all the centers.

At the St. Jude Children's Research Hospital in Memphis, Tennessee, nearly all ALL treatments are done on an out-patient basis. The children stay at homes and in nerby motels, and come in regularly to be treated. This in no way reduces the effectiveness of the treatment. In fact, Dr. Joseph V. Simone, the hospital's Chief of Hematology points out that "in addition to making children and parents happier, out-patient care reduces exposure to other diseases being treated in the hospital and permits the hospital's staff to care for more children."

Dr. Simone uses the full range of latest chemotherapy techniques as well as irradiation of the brain aimed at preventing a relapse of the disease. The actual treatment includes first an intensive program of powerful drugs—including direct injections into the spinal column—and continued treatment with smaller doses for an indefinite period.

This follow-up is very important because if the disease returns, chances of success with another round of treatment are greatly reduced. "Each child with ALL needs a personal physician to look after him," says Dr. Simone. "To be prepared, the physician who decides to care for the child with

ALL must work with a modern cancer center, collaborate with a center or obtain appropriate experience there before assuming that responsibility." St. Jude's cooperates fully and widely with local physicians caring for the children after their initial treatment at the center.

Information on the location of your nearest specialized ALL treatment center can be obtained from;

National Cancer Institute
Building 10
Bethesda, Md. 20014

40. CEMENTING ARTIFICIAL HIP JOINTS

AN OLD DENTAL CEMENT, adapted many years ago by dentists for sealing dentures and bridges, is now being used for cementing artificial hip joints. The cement—*methyl methacrylate*—has been used in hip surgery in Europe for over 12 years, but has been approved for use in this country only since 1971.

Artificial hip joints are used to relieve persons with deteriorated hips caused by arthritis. An arthritic hip joint loses its smooth working surfaces, becoming rough, inflamed, and painful. To relieve this condition, surgeons have been implanting artificial, metal ball-and-socket joints which are installed after the diseased bone has been removed. These screwed-in joints have various disadvantages. One problem is that they are smaller than natural hip joints and impede the natural action of the hip muscles. Another problem is friction. This friction, generated by the metal-to-metal joint, creates an increased torque force which loosens the entire apparatus.

To reduce the friction, a British surgeon, Dr. John Charnley, developed a socket of acrylic plastic which is fitted against a ball fashioned from a cobalt-chrome alloy. To replace the old, slow, unsatisfactory method of fixing the artificial hip joint in place, Dr. Charnley used the cement,

---

Additional material touching on this subject can be found in chapters 6, 18 and 80.

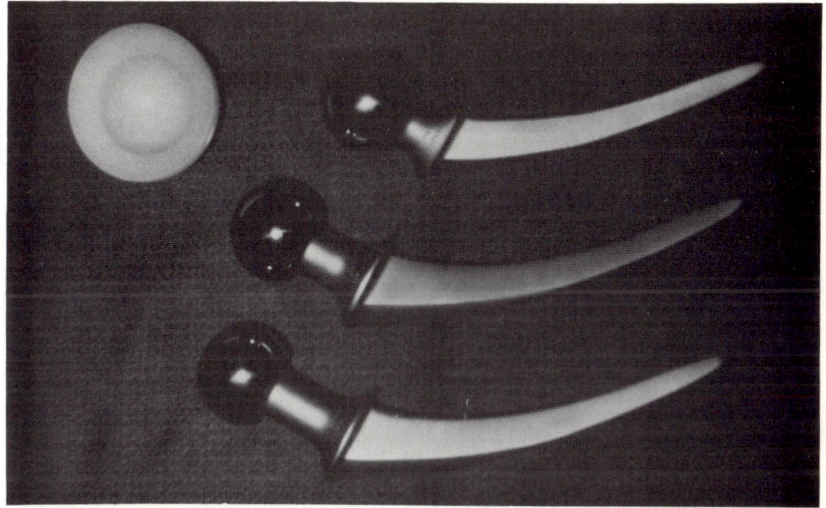

Components of artificial hip joints. a plastic socket and several ball-and-stem units in various sizes. The plastic socket fits in the pelvic bone, and the metal ball and stem fits in the femoral shaft.

which is molded into shape and hardens quickly and permanently.

The use of the cement prevents the artificial joints from working themselves loose in the bone and it allows the use of natural-sized artificial joints that distribute the person's weight over a larger area of the hip socket than the smaller, screw-in devices. This permits more natural action of the hip muscles.

The greatest advantage of the new procedure is almost immediate freedom from pain, since there is no rubbing of bone against bone in the hip joint. Many persons have suffered incapacitating pain for years and have found no relief until now.

Other advantages of this operation are that the patient can stand and start walking much sooner than under the old procedure; a relatively short period of hospitalization and fairly short convalescence. There are no casts. The heavy muscles which surround the implant help secure it.

41. GIVING VOICE
TO LARYNGECTOMEES

LARYNGECTOMEES—persons whose larynx has been removed and who are able to speak with a natural-sounding voice are rare. Once a person has had his larynx (voice box) removed, he must learn what is called esophageal speech; he must use an outside type of artificial larynx; or he must remain silent.

Most persons who must have their larynx removed undergo the operation after having incurred cancer of the larynx. According to the American Cancer Society, there are more than 25,000 laryngectomees—persons with a removed larynx—in the U S., and an additional 3,800 will be added to this group this year.

About one-third of these patients are *unable* to learn the esophageal speech method. This is a long process of training with the assistance of a speech specialist whereby the patient is taught to bring the voice up from the stomach. They have to use artificial larynx devices—electronic resonators—instruments which are held up to the neck and assist the patient in speaking with varying degrees of success.

But many laryngectomees are unable to master either the difficult esophageal speech or the electronic devices. These people are condemned to a life of silence.

Now, thanks to the ingenuity of a New York Medical

Additional material touching on this subject can be found in chapters 5 and 78.

College surgeon, Dr. Stanley Taub, these silent laryngectomees can have their speech immediately restored with a
device which he recently invented.

The beauty of the device, which is called VoiceBak, is that
it requires no training of any kind. It works immediately—the
instant it is put on. Many of the laryngectomees who have
used it were able to sing, shout or whisper, and even to count
to twenty on a single breath.

The VoiceBak is a specially designed set of valve
mechanisms made of light plastic. It is invisible when worn
under a tie and shirt or under a high-neck dress or a scarf.

In order to be able to wear the VoiceBak, the laryngec-
tomee has to have an operation called a *modified cervical es-
ophagostomy*. The device is fitted to the patient by the surgeon in accordance with a procedure introduced by Dr. Taub.

Despite its long medical name, the operation is only the formation of an opening in the neck, carefully executed in the
patient's esophagus. The surgeon makes a cut in the patient's
neck and creates a skin-lined tube from his esophagus to the
side of his neck, a short distance and slightly higher from the
opening in the throat left by the removal of the larynx. Usually, this second opening is made on the left side of the neck.

In order to qualify for the operation the patient must be
free of recurrent cancer, and must have positive psychologic
motivation for the operation.

Once the operation has been performed, three weeks are
allowed for healing and then the patient is fitted with the
VoiceBak. The device doesn't contain any electronic or electrical parts, but works mechanically, using the laryngec-
tomee's own respiratory system. It does not interfere with
eating or drinking, and can be worn all day. At night, it is
easily removed and is just as easily replaced in the morning.
(A tube with a special plug on the end is used at night to block
the newly created opening in the neck.)

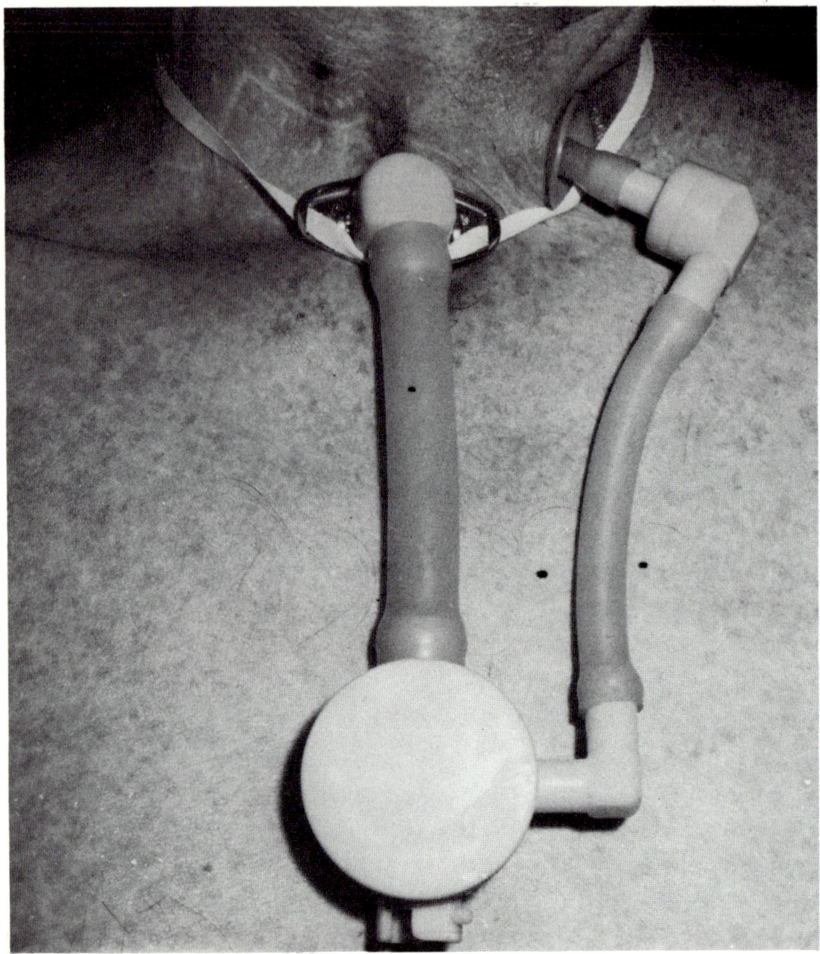

The Voice Bak Prosthesis as it is normally worn. At the top, on the right side of the picture, the fistula valve can be seen connected to the surgically-made opening in the side of the neck.

VoiceBak weighs only three ounces and its unique feature is that it provides speech that has natural regional and ethnic accents. It is made by LaBarge, Inc., of St. Louis, Missouri, and is sold only to physicians (presently, at $950). It is available for immediate delivery.

42. A LASER "KNIFE" FOR BLOODLESS SURGERY

SURGEONS TODAY have a new type of "knife" at their disposal: the laser. The laser is an instrument which produces a beam of light of such tremendous energy and power that its light is a million times as intense as at the surface of the sun.

This beam of light can be flashed through a lens which causes the beam to be "squeezed together" into a light beam that ends as a tiny, brilliant spot on the other side of the lens. This spot may be smaller than the point of a pin, and is so hot that it will "drill" (by melting) a hole into any metal.

Laser beams have various uses in medicine today, both in treatment and as instrumentation for diagnosis. The most interesting use right now is in surgery. Because there is no bleeding in certain forms of laser surgery (the heat of the beam coagulates the blood) it is used in various medical procedures where bleeding is of great concern. A laser unit at the Medical Center of the University of Cincinnati has been used for removal of burns and, because of bloodless surgery, immediate skin graft replacement.

Laser beams are also used to clean up the skin by burning out small or large warts, birthmarks and tattoos. The laser laboratory of the Children's Hospital Research Foundation of the Medical Center of the University of Cincinnati is one of

---

Additional material touching on this subject can be found in chapter 70.

the first and largest laser research centers. Its director, Dr. Leon Goldman, a pioneer in laser medicine, has become involved in juvenile delinquency rehabilitation programs because he can remove certain types of youngsters' tattoos with his lasers.

Dr. Goldman is also experimenting with the laser in the diagnosis of cancer of the breast. This procedure (using harmless beams) is called laser *transillumination* and is based on detection of various densities of body tissues.

Laser is widely used in eye surgery. It is used to repair damage to the retina. One common condition is a retina which has pulled away from the eye wall behind it. To repair it, the surgeon shoots a laser beam into the eye. The beam passes through the transparent front part of the eye, hits the solid retina, and welds it to the eye wall behind it.

The .retina may be damaged in other ways. It might be punctured or torn, and these damages are repaired with the laser beam which seals them to keep them from spreading.

In another eye condition, a membrane—called pterygium —forms, covering the eye and causing blindness. Since this membrane is fed by enlarged veins, conventional surgery is impossible because of the threat of hemorrhage. With the laser, the surgeon cuts through the membrane, then seals the end of the veins where the ''cut'' was made. With the veins sealed, the blood supply is cut off and the membrane cannot grow back.

A type of laser called the *Argon Laser* is widely used in treatment of diabetes of the eye. This kind of laser beam can be pinpointed so precisely that it will hit a spot half the thickness of a human hair. Because of this, it can be used safely no matter how close to vital organs. The procedure is called *argon laser photocoagulation,* and it involves the use of the beam to eliminate newly formed blood vessels in the eye which bleed causing diabetic blindness.

Dr. Goldman finds the laser a valuable tool in fighting cancer. It can be used through a microscope to focus down to a point 1/25,000 of an inch in diameter. Tiny holes can be drilled into red blood corpuscles and the contents of the cancerous cells destroyed without damaging the surrounding membranes in tissue cultures. Closed circuit television makes it possible to fire a laser at active moving cells while watching them. The laser, especially laser called CO_2, can be used through a microscope for treatment of certain forms of cancer of the throat and other organs.

Dr. Goldman predicts an important future for this new "knife" (first used in 1960). He has already used laser knives to perform bloodless spleen and liver surgery on experimental animals.

43. HAIR TRANSPLANTATION

THOUGH MANY MEN do not believe that it is possible to grow hair on a bald pate, the medical fact is that hair transplantation is now an accepted surgical procedure. The doctor responsible for this acceptance is Dr. Norman Orentreich, of New York City, whose "punch graft" transplantation technique is considered the best way to grow hair on a person who is bald.

Dr. Orentreich's procedure—medically called *scalp punch autografts*—involves transplanting hair from that part of the head which still has some hair left, to the bald section. A new hairline is formed and the transplanted hair grows in naturally, covering the baldness.

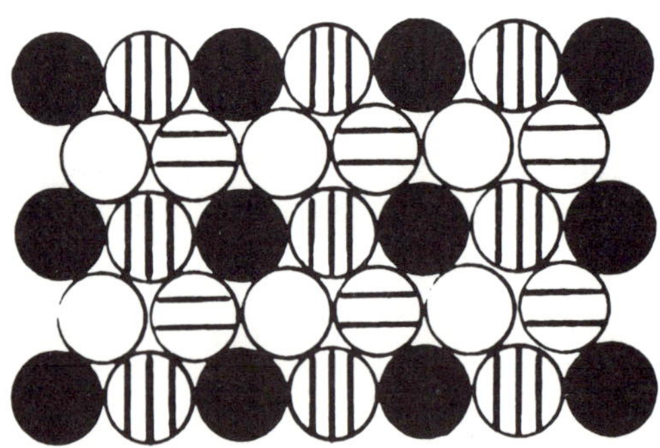

Scalp grafts are separated by the width of the punch diameter. Four procedures are necessary to completely fill in an area.

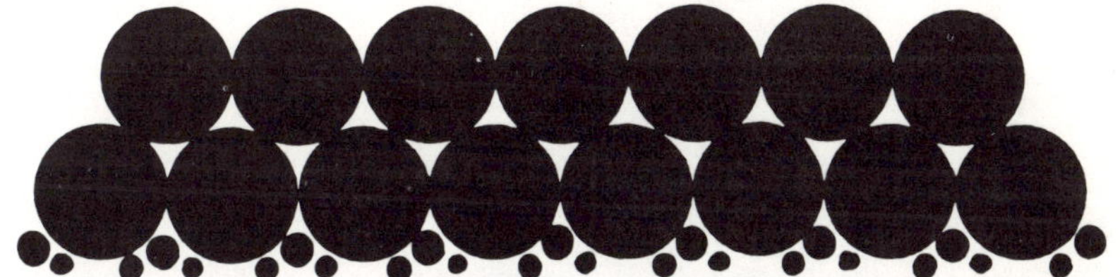

Smaller grafts are used to create a more natural hairline.

Though the transplant technique is a simple procedure from the point of view of a surgeon, nevertheless, it requires a considerable degree of knowledge and skill. If performed incorrectly, the transplanted hair may not grow out, or, even worse, it may grow in the wrong direction. It may grow in a direction opposite to that of the natural hair that is on the scalp and that had not fallen out.

Inept surgeons have been known to create unnatural hairlines—straight across, arched or pointed. Thus, hair transplantation, although a simple procedure, is best left to specialists, many of whom are members of the American Society for Dermatologic Surgery. (This society, located at 1150 North West 14th Street, Miami, Florida, can advise interested readers of the addresses of specialists in their vicinity.)

Even though hair transplantation is done in the doctor's office under local anesthesia, it is a surgical procedure with considerable post-operative pain and discomfort, and a man must have the required degree of determination to go through the procedure.

Today's transplantation technique involves the use of a special punch, created by Dr. Orentreich. Using this punch, the surgeon removes small plugs of skin with hair attached from one part of the head and transplants them into holes previously punched out with the punch in the area designated to be covered with the new hairgrowth. The number of transplants depends on the area of baldness to be covered,

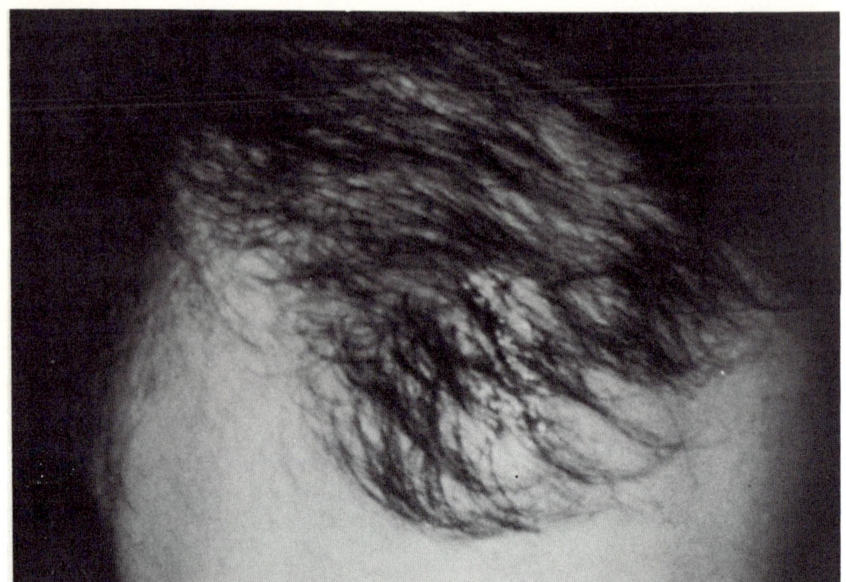

The front of the scalp, showing multiple grafts, one to four months after transplantation.

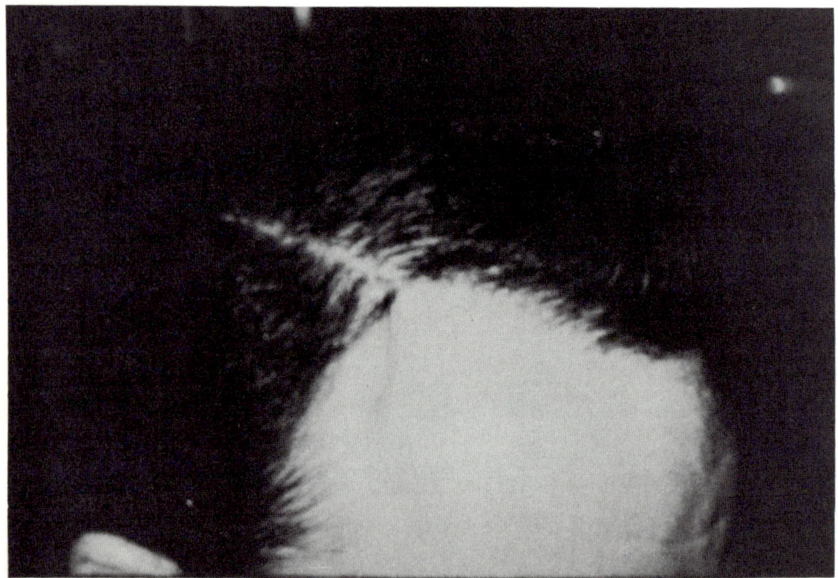

Two years later, the frontal scalp grafting shows a vigorous full growth of hair.

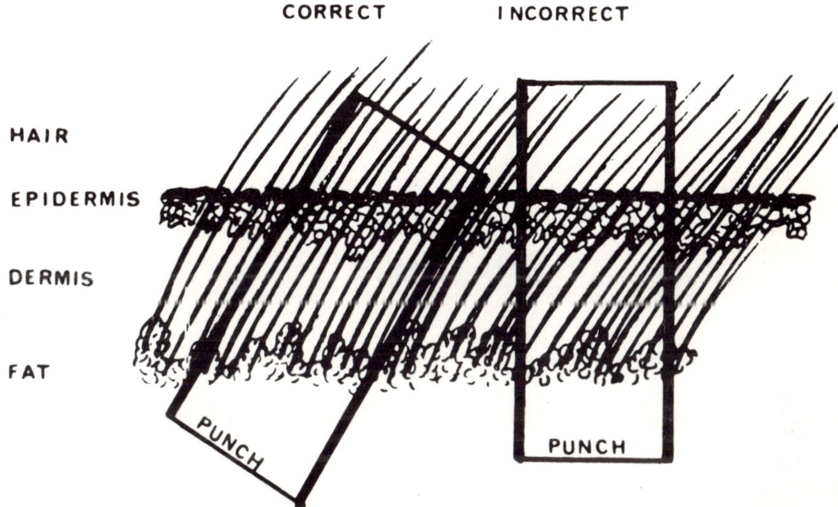

The correct and incorrect angles for cutting donor plugs. The average 4mm. plug contains 12 to 15 hairs. The transplanted hair does not start to grow until three months after the transplantation.

availability of hair for transplanting, and the tolerance of the patient to the procedure.

The average number of transplanted plugs is 200 to 300, with 10 to 50 being grafted during each session. Dr. Orentreich believes that the smaller number of plugs per session is better as the smaller area is quicker to "take" and the chances of its becoming a healthy growth of hair are improved. At least two weeks must be allowed for healing, between sessions.

The current costs range from $5 to $25 per plug transplanted, with the total cost ranging from $300 to $1,000 depending on the needs and desires of the patient.

44. HEART MEDICATION CAN CONTROL TREMORS

TREMORS, OR INVOLUNTARY MOVEMENTS, can have many causes, including thyroid and nervous-system disease, anxiety states, palpitation of the heart, chronic mercury poisoning, poisoning by lead, zinc or other metals, alcoholism, and opium addiction. But in some cases, the tremors are called "essential," because no cause can be found.

Essential tremor appears when a hand is used for a particular task, especially one which requires careful attention (such as writing, or carrying a cup filled with liquid). The tremor can be severe enough to disrupt a person's work and to interfere with the carrying out of normal social activities. It is particularly frustrating because as soon as the hand is rested, the tremor stops; only to return as soon as a new attempt is made to use the hand.

Until now, the only effective medication was alcohol, but it is only effective for a short period of time after taking a drink. In addition, there is always the danger of becoming an alcoholic or suffering from various side-effects produced by the consumption of alcohol.

Now, a drug previously used to control abnormal heart rhythm was found to control the essential tremors. The discovery was made by Dr. Gerald F. Winkler, of the Massachusetts General Hospital in Boston. Its usefulness was discovered when Dr. Winkler treated a woman suffering from such severe tremors that she had not been able to sign her name during the last five years. She developed an abnormal heart rhythm for which her doctor gave her a drug called Propranolol. Dr. Winkler noticed that the drug not only controlled her heartbeat—but that her tremors disappeared!

In collaboration with Dr. Robert Young, Dr. Winkler immediately set up study groups. He has since reported that 80% of the tested patients with severe tremors have shown good or excellent improvement. None of the tested patients was worse. Several of the patients continued the medication on a long-term basis, and more than a year after they started, showed that they continued to benefit from the drug.

The new treatment does not produce any serious side-effects or discomfort, but Propranolol cannot be given to persons suffering from congestive heart failure, asthma, and certain other allergic disorders.

The dosage required is adjusted to the individual need of each patient, and it is not necessary to drug him so heavily as to stop the tremors completely. It is enough to reduce the strength of the tremors to the point where they no longer interfere with writing, eating, or other activities of daily living. It was found that a mild shaking was quite acceptable to those who previously suffered severe tremors.

Not the least important point of the new discovery is the fact that treatment with Propranolol is within the financial reach of the majority of sufferers from essential tremors.

45. QUICK TEST
FOR CHILDHOOD CANCER

NEUROBLASTOMA is a highly malignant cancer that is one of the most common causes of death in small children. The disease begins as a tiny, solid tumor. If it can be removed by surgery at that stage, 80% of the patients can be cured. However, once the tumor begins to metastasize—spread through the body—the chances of survival grow dim.

More than 90% of the children die if the cancer spreads by the time it is detected. Even if the tumors are only 50% metastasized the chances of survival are less than 50%.

Obviously, as with all cancers, the sooner the doctor can start treatment, the better the chances. Unfortunately, neuroblastoma is very difficult to spot. Too often, the condition is not discovered until the mother feels a lump on the baby's neck or stomach. By then, it is often too late.

Now, a new, quick and cheap test for early detection of most cases has been discovered, according to Dr. Arnold S. Leonard, chief of pediatric surgery at the University of Minnesota Medical School in Minneapolis.

The test is based on the fact that up to 80% of the childhood neuroblastoma tumors excrete a substance called *3-methoxy 4-hydroxy mandelic acid* (VMA). This VMA shows up in the child's urine.

Additional material touching on this subject can be found in chapters 17 and 39.

The new test is simple: If a strip of paper treated with special chemicals is dipped into the urine—or just pressed against a wet diaper—it will change color if VMA is present. The "dip stick" strips come pre-packaged and cost less than 15 cents each.

The new test strips will make it simple and inexpensive for doctors to test all children for neuroblastoma as part of the periodic examination routine. Dr. Leonard says that testing should be done every other month for the first year of a child's life, every four months until the child is two years old, and twice yearly thereafter, until the age of ten.

The University of Minnesota hospitals and other health care centers are now using the strip test for routine, mass screening of all children under seven years of age. Many individual physicians have also begun using the test on all their young patients. Dr. Leonard is optimistic that in time the test will become a standard part of all baby examinations.

46. RESPIRATORY PACEMAKER: A MECHANICAL AID TO BREATHING

A QUADRIPLEGIC with respiratory paralysis has been able to breathe without the aid of a *mechanical respirator* for more than a year. He has been using a new device called a *diaphragm pacemaker* which was developed by Dr. William W. L. Glenn of the Yale University School of Medicine.

Also, eight patients suffering from severe *Ondin's Curse* [inability to breathe properly because of malfunction of the phrenic (diaphragm) nerve] have been greatly helped with the implantation of this new device. Several of them were able to return to normal activities.

Persons suffering from this malady, and quadriplegics with respiratory paralysis, are desperately in need of one or another of the various available mechanical aids in order to help them breathe. Ondin's Curse sufferers need this help at night, during sleep, when they literally forget to breathe and have to use iron lungs, tank respirators, rocking beds and various other devices of this nature to keep breathing while they sleep. Quadriplegics require continuous mechanical breathing aid.

The new diaphragm pacemaker makes mechanical aids unnecessary. It works by stimulating the phrenic nerve, which causes the diaphragm to descend, pulling air into the lungs. The device, adapted from an ordinary heart pacemaker, uses

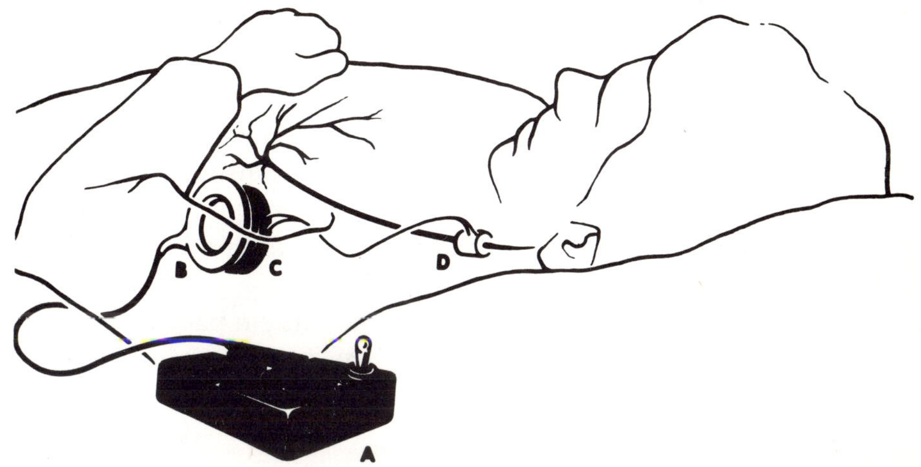

The electrophrenic respiration apparatus includes a battery-run transmitter (A) which transmits radio frequency signals through the antenna (B) to the implanted receiver (C). The implanted receiver is connected by wires under the skin to the implanted cuff (D) surrounding the phrenic nerve.

radio waves to stimulate the phrenic nerve and induce "electrophrenic respiration" (ERP).

In the actual operation, which is performed under local anesthesia, Dr. Glenn exposes the phrenic nerve—which is easily reached. He simply makes a small incision, and encircles it with an electrode connected with a wire laid under the skin, to a receiver which he implants under the skin over the ribs. The incision is then closed, and an antenna is taped to the skin over the implanted receiver. The patient is supplied with a pocket-size transmitter which emits radio-frequency (RF) signals. The receiver changes the RF into electrical impulses, which stimulate the phrenic nerve.

In implanting the diaphragm pacemaker in patients with Ondin's Curse, Dr. Glenn uses the left phrenic nerve (there is one on each side of the body). In the case of the quadriplegic with respiratory paralysis, single nerve stimulation didn't work out because the stimulation had to be constant, while in cases of Ondin's Curse it is only needed at night.

Twelve hours is the limit of time that one phrenic nerve can be stimulated with RF, and this was a problem. The problem was solved by Dr. Glenn by implanting electrodes around both nerves, implanting two receivers, one on each side of the body, and sending out an RF from the transmitter which stimulated the nerves on an alternate basis: First the left nerve 12 hours, then the right nerve 12 hours, and back again to the left nerve, and so on.

Dr. Glenn has now implanted the diaphragm pacemaker in a second quadriplegic patient, and he is making excellent progress adapting to it.

47. ORTHOKERATOLOGY

THIS MEDICAL TONGUE-TWISTER is the name of a new technique that may reduce myopia (nearsightedness) for some persons.

With myopia, the eyeball is longer than it should be. Light rays, bending at a normal angle as they enter the eye, come to focus in front of the retina instead of on it. A myopic or near-sighted person sees near objects clearly, but distant objects are usually blurred.

Orthokeratology is defined as reduction modification or elimination of a visual defect by the programmed application of contact lenses or other related procedures. In actual prac-tice, researchers in orthokeratology prescribe special contact lenses to change the curvature of the cornea (exterior surface of the eye).

According to Dr. Bertrand A. Kolles, an orthokeratology specialist of St. Paul, Minnesota, there are two basic ap-proaches to the care of myopia with the new technique. In one, the optometrist prescribes a corrective contact lens with refractive power (that is, such as improve the vision). The patient's eyes are tested at intervals and when it is determined that the maximum change in the curvature of the cornea has been obtained with these lenses, new lenses with a different

---

Additional material touching on this subject can be found in chapters 35 and 56.

power are prescribed. This maximum change may occur in as little time as three weeks or as long as three months. The other approach involves prescribing contact lenses with no refractive power and altering the wearing time to bring about the desired changes in the curvature of the cornea and the resulting reduction of the refractive error and improvement of the unaided visual acuity.

Orthokeratology usually involves many visits by the patient to the optometrist's office for observation of the lens fit and of any changes in the shape of the cornea. The results obtained by the optometric researchers indicate that orthokeratology is safe and effective in treating or reducing myopia in persons of any age, although not everyone can benefit from the procedures.

According to Dr. Reid H. Anderson, an ophthalmologist in Idaho Falls, Idaho, myopia can be arrested (its progress halted) and/or controlled by use of contact lenses. In a study of 170 eyes with 3,800 months of wearing time, Dr. Anderson found that the progress of myopia—deterioration of vision—was 27 times as great in those wearing glasses than in those wearing contacts.

Many contact lenses prescribed today are sold with "lifetime guarantee," or "once you wear contact lenses you'll never need to change them" concept. According to Dr. Charles May, an orthokeratology specialist in San Diego, California, these concepts are not sound. He believes that orthokeratology is the proper approach to long-range contact lens fitting techniques, and that its method of prescribing new lenses at intervals benefits the patient vision. Since, despite the "guarantees," the life expectancy of a pair of contact lenses is limited—they do get lost, or stepped on when they fall on the floor—the idea of having new lenses prescribed at intervals may not necessarily result in having many more pairs of contacts made than if one were to duplicate the original prescription when a new pair of contacts is needed.

With those who are helped, it has been found that some persons, after experiencing orthokeratology techniques, have been able to go without corrective lenses for as long as three years, while others need retainer type contact lenses on a periodic basis for short intervals. "Retainer contacts" are contact lenses used to maintain the improved vision after successful achievement of the desired change. If contact lenses are discontinued too quickly after reaching 20/20 unaided vision, the person may lose some acuity, and that is why his wearing schedule must be reduced slowly over several months.

Specific fitting procedures have been devised for the new technique, which is based on programmed follow-up care which requires changes in the lens design. Not all optometrists use the new technique, but the International Orthokeratology Society, 6505 Alvardo Road, San Diego, California 92120, can furnish the names of its members located near any readers who may be interested in investigating the new technique for his or her personal benefit.

48. MIGRAINE—
PROMISING NEW AID

A RECENTLY-INTRODUCED drug for abnormal heart rhythms—propranolol—was discovered to be a "safe and effective treatment" in cases of severe migraine.

Recently, doctors noted an improvement in headaches of patients being treated with propranolol for heart disease. Now, a study of 19 patients with severe migraines, conducted by Dr. Oscar M. Reinmuth and Dr. Ronald B. Weber of the University of Miami, confirmed that the new drug is not only effective in treatment of migraine, but, according to Dr. Reinmuth, "it may be the drug of choice for individuals who, because of various medical reasons, cannot use Ergot or Methysergide (the two top migraine remedies)."

The drug is also an effective treatment, where the two remedies just mentioned have failed to provide relief.

During the study, all patients were given propranolol some of the time, and a placebo (a look-alike, no-effect preparation) the rest of the time. It was what the doctors call a double-blind study, which means that neither the patient nor the physician knew when the real drug or the placebo was being used until after the study was over.

Fifteen of the 19 patients had a 50% or better reduction in the frequency or severity of the headaches, and of those, six

---

Additional material touching on this subject can be found in chapters 57, 67, 79, 85 and 91.

reported that all, or almost all, headaches disappeared after the first week on propranolol.

Dr. Reinmuth is continuing the use of propranolol in treatment of migraine, with "worthwhile" success. In some individuals, reports Dr. Reinmuth, propranolol is successful when taken at the onset of the headache. "The majority of the patients that I see," he remarked, "have had treatment failure with standard Ergot and Methysergide regimens. A significant number of these are able to obtain relief with moderate doses of propranolol, taken two or three times a day."

Dr. Reinmuth believes that propranolol is definitely a better method of migraine treatment than the large number of undefined "last line of defense" treatments now being employed.

49. VITAMINS FOR INTERMITTENT CLAUDICATION

INTERMITTENT CLAUDICATION IS a condition which manifests itself in a temporary loss of function in the heart or brain, and is caused by spasm in the artery.

The condition is often caused by an artery in the leg called the *femoral artery*. The condition can become so bad that the artery turns into a gristly cord, and the pain, caused by the blockage of the blood supply to the leg, becomes so intense as to make walking impossible.

Surgical procedures are often required, but they involve some deaths and may cause serious after-effects. Also, intermittent claudication may be caused by blockage of small arteries in or below the knee, in which cases surgical treatment is of uncertain benefit. It is used only as a last resort to attempt to relieve the person of unbearable pain.

A team of physicians led by Dr. H. T. G. Williams of the University of Alberta Hospital at Edmonton, Canada, has found vitamin E to be successful in the treatment of intermittent claudication.

The vitamin E treatment tried by Dr. Williams involved a group of 45 patients. Each received (by mouth) 400mg doses of vitamin E four times a day for three months.

This group of patients suffered from intermittent claudication caused by blockage of arteries in various locations in the body (the leg arteries are not the only ones which cause this condition). The results showed that those patients with the condition caused by diseased arteries in the legs were the ones who benefited from the vitamin E treatment, while the treatment had little, or no effect on those whose disease was caused by blockage of arteries in other parts of the body.

Dr. Williams' current study was actually a culmination of a 10-year study on the use of vitamin E to relieve this condition. He is now convinced that vitamin E has a definite place in the treatment of intermittent claudication.

50. REGAINING FERTILITY VIA MICROSURGERY

LIGATION OF FALLOPIAN TUBES—surgical closing of the tubes—is becoming more and more the choice of many women who want to insure against conception. They find that other means of contraception are either less effective, more troublesome, or require too high a degree of sustained motivation.

But many women who undergo tubal ligation remarry and decide that they want a child. They become as dedicated to the goal of regaining their fertility as they were before in preventing it.

Medically, tubal ligation is considered an irreversible procedure. Once performed, it is final. Attempts at reversal have proven to be very difficult and the results very uncertain.

Now, a Philadelphia surgeon, Dr. Celso-Ramon Garcia, of the University of Pennsylvania, has reported having successfully performed a reverse tubal ligation in seven out of 14 patients, with three patients subsequently reporting four pregnancies.

Dr. Garcia attributes much of his success to his use of microsurgery. Using an operating microscope in working on the very fine tubes has many advantages and eliminates the

---

Additional material touching on this subject can be found in chapter 55.

possibility of closing a tube further, instead of repairing it. "Putting a stitch into the tissue with the naked eye," explains Dr. Garcia, "you not only grab the one wall, but you may take with it a piece of the opposite wall, which means that in fact you're closing it up instead of trying to repair it."

The immediate objective of a ligation reversal procedure is to achieve *patency*—a condition of being freely opened. This has been achieved in all seven successful reversals, and this patency rate of 50% is better than in most other reversal operations performed with the naked eye. Conception, according to Dr. Garcia, can take a year or two, as the tubes gradually return to normal functioning. All four of the pregnancies of his patients occurred more than six months after the reversal operations, and they were uncomplicated. The woman who has had two pregnancies has delivered full-term babies both times.

Dr. Garcia does not consider that his 50% success rate is absolute proof that microsurgery is an improvement over naked eye operations, but he does belive that it is definitely the superior method for achieving patency. "X-rays tell us that the tubes are perfectly normal," says Dr. Garcia. "You can't tell there has been a disruption."

51. SURGERY FOR HYDROCEPHALIC INFANTS

IT IS WELL KNOWN to doctors that a large number of *hydrocephalic* children—infants with "water on the brain"—require no medical treatment at all. In fact, many children with this condition are probably never identified correctly as having it.

Infantile hydrocephalus is a condition which is usually present at birth. It is caused by a heavy discharge of a clear, watery fluid from blood vessels, called *cerebro spinal fluid (CSF)*, into the *cerebral ventricles*—the brain sections inside the skull.

The accumulating CSF dilates these ventricles, thinning the brain and causing a separation of the bones in the skull by an increase of intracranial pressure. The head becomes enlarged and the child afflicted often becomes mentally retarded.

In some cases, no treatment is necessary—the CSF might be absorbed by the body. But, in other cases, immediate surgery is required. Without treatment, the progress of the disease can change for better or for worse. The big problem facing a doctor examining hydrocephalic children lies in separating those who can be expected to recover without treatment, from those who require surgery.

If the accumulation of a CSF is caused by a tumor in the skull or the narrowing of the canal that normally carries away a natural accumulation of CSF, this can be easily detected by the doctor and surgery can promptly relieve the condition.

However, when the reason for the accumulation of the serum cannot be determined by examination, the surgeon must operate and insert into the skull a device called a *shunt*. The shunt is a pump which removes the accumulated serum and injects it into the blood stream. Once the child is shunted —as the procedure is called—he becomes shunt-dependent and even if the CSF accumulation subsides he must continue to use the shunt. Because of this, many children who originally didn't need the shunt at all end up shunt-dependent.

A team of Austrian physicians at the University of Graz, led by Dr. Ian Knoetgen of the Graz Neurosurgery Clinic, developed a new technique that tells the surgeon when an operation is unnecessary—information that could substantially reduce the number of hydrocephalus operations. Not only does it prevent needless surgery, but it also avoids insertion of shunts in certain borderline patients who would become shunt-dependent if the operation were to be performed.

Dr. Knoetgen's technique involves the use of a radioisotope, and taking certain measurements as the radioisotope works its way through the body. The radioisotope, called ^{131}I-hippuran, is injected into the cerebral ventricle and its transfer into the patient's blood is traced by special detectors. The procedure is painless and takes from 30 minutes to an hour.

The information picked up by the detector is fed to a high-speed printer and becomes available to the doctor in the form of printed charts. By comparing the results of the tracing shown on the chart, with tables prepared by Dr. Knoetgen, the surgeon can determine if the child needs immediate surgery or whether there is a good possibility of self-recovery.

According to Dr. Knoetgen, between 40% and 46% of hydrocephalic patients can recover without surgery.

52. PERITONEAL DIALYSIS AT HOME FOR JUST $20

PERSONS WITHOUT KIDNEYS must undergo dialysis—have their blood cleansed of impurities by a machine, which takes the place of the kidneys and removes the impurities from the blood. Without the machine, impurities build up in the bloodstream and the person dies, poisoned by his own urine.

For a long time cost has blocked the way to home *hemodialysis*. Now, Dr. Norman Lasker, of the Jefferson Medical College in Philadelphia, has developed a home *peritoneal dialysis* unit, which not only solves many technical problems, but brings most of the benefits of an artificial kidney at a substantially reduced cost.

In hemodialysis, the patient's blood flows from the body to a machine which cleanses the blood by passing it through a coil immersed in a chemical bath. Impurities, such as urea, flow from the blood into the chemicals through a membrane in the coil, and the cleansed blood is pumped back into the patient's veins. In peritoneal dialysis no outside blood washing machine is used, but the peritoneal (abdomen) lining is the filter through which the body wastes are passed out into the dialyzing solution (chemical bath) and then drained from the body through an abdominal catheter. Dr. Lasker's dialysis unit is combined with an *indwelling* (permanently placed in) *catheter* which can remain fixed in the abdomen for many

Additional material touching on this subject can be found in chapters 54 and 88.

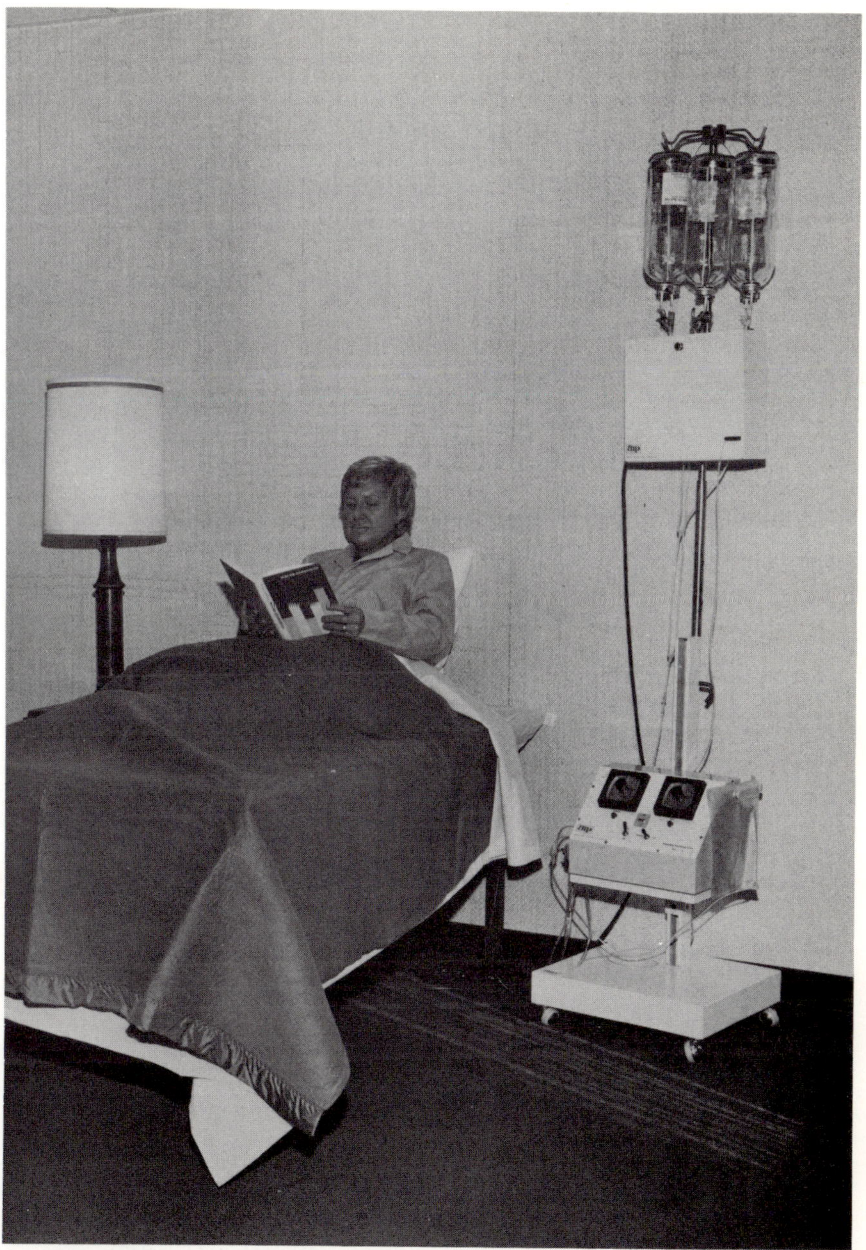

The Automatic Peritoneal Cycler in use in the dialysis unit of the Jefferson Medical College.

months and possibly years.

The new unit, manufactured by the American Medical Products Corp., of Fairfield, New Jersey, can be used in a hospital but is primarily designed for home dialysis where the patient can use it at night while he sleeps.

The machine is completely portable and is so simple and safe that it can be operated by the user without any outside help. A built-in drain alarm warns in the event that the patient is not draining properly.

According to Dr. Lasker, learning to use the machine takes two to three weeks, as compared with about two months for hemodialysis.

Peritoneal dialysis may be done twice a week as against thrice weekly hemodialysis. The new unit uses 10 or 20-liter (one liter is slightly over one quart) plastic containers of *dialysate* (dialyzing solution) as compared with the conventional one or two-liter bottles. Since 40 liters are needed for a single dialysis, only two hookups are needed instead of the previous minimum of 20. This greatly cuts the risk of infection. The use of the large fluid containers and the unit's automatic cycler have reduced the time needed for a single dialysis from 20 hours to 11—thus only 22 hours are needed each week for the procedure. This is not much more than the 18 hours weekly required for three hemodialysis sessions.

A single dialysis with Dr. Lasker's unit costs under $20 as against $170 for an in-hospital peritoneal dialysis. This takes into consideration that the present cost of the dialysate is about sixty cents per liter. There are good prospects, however, that this cost can be brought down by the manufacturers to around twenty-five cents. The machine costs $1,500, including an optional lift unit ($250) for raising the dialyzing solution to the desired height and providing a movable stand for the cycler.

53. SIDESTEPPING SURGERY FOR UNDESCENDED TESTICLES

UNDESCENDED TESTICLES are a major psychological problem for the affected child. How soon or how late to operate to correct this problem has been an open question. Some doctors operate on infants—others wait until the onset of puberty, and beyond.

According to Dr. John K. Lattimer, Professor and Chief of Urology at Columbia University College of Physicians and Surgeons, in New York City, treatment with hormones may make surgery unnecessary.

Side effects of hormone injections are minor and have not been reported to be objectionable either by the parents or by the child. There is some increase in the size of the penis and some pubic fuzz appears during the course of the injections. The chance of correcting an undescended testicle on one side are about 15%, says Dr. Lattimer. If both testicles are un-descended—a condition medically called bilateral cryp-torchism—the chances of success with hormone treatments are better than 30%.

Dr. Lattimer believes that if the surgery is necessary, it should be done before the child's sixth birthday, because if the testicles are not brought down into the scrotum by this age, but are left up in the body, they may be damaged by internal body heat.

By the time boys are five, says Dr. Lattimer, they often start

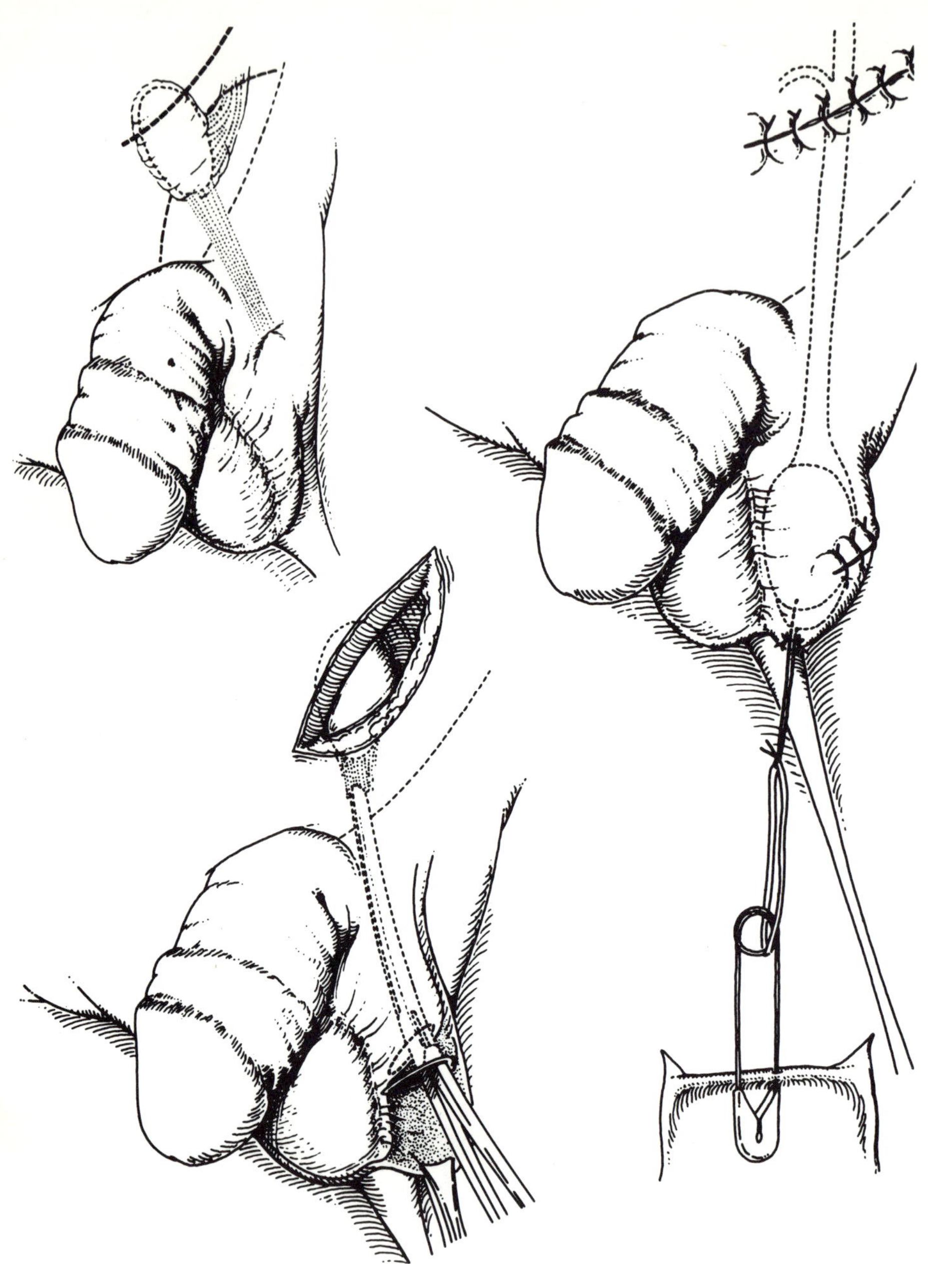

An operation for an undescended testicle. First, a curved transverse incision is outlined and then made in the skin fold (top, left). The testis is then pulled through the scrotum and out the scrotal "window" (bottom, left). To complete the procedure, the traction suture is tied to a small rubber band (right) which is pinned with a large safety pin to a band of adhesive just above the knee of the opposite leg. The tension of the rubber band is just enough to prevent the traction suture from drooping.

comparing genitals and worry about anything unusual, such as an empty scrotal sac. Therefore, he favors starting the hormone treatments between the fourth and fifth birthdays.

"Migratory testis"—a condition in which the testicles "travel up and down," sometimes being up in the body and at other times in the scrotum—is seldom treated. Usually, the traveling testicles settle permanently in the scrotum by the age of puberty. However, such a testicle which suddenly disappears without a reason can cause the boy unnecessary psychological agonies and might result in permanent emotional problems.

Because the testicles do, in the end, settle in the scrotum, many doctors and parents don't consider this a serious condition and no treatment is given. "This," says Dr. Lattimer, "is wrong. Treatment is always indicated to avoid potential emotional damage to the boy."

Dr. Lattimer gives the child three injections of gonadotropic hormone, one every other day, and this is usually enough to bring the migratory testicles down, which proves to the child that there is nothing to worry about.

54. KIDNEY TRANSPLANTS FOR DIABETICS

DIABETES MELLITUS, commonly called *diabetes*, is a disease characterized by too much sugar in the blood. Two of its symptoms are excessive urination and great thirst. When the sugar in the blood reaches a certain level, some of it is excreted by the kidneys in urine. This causes frequent urination and also causes the afflicted to develop a great thirst, leading to drinking enormous quantities of water and further heavy urination. Because of the burning thirst, when the disease was first described in medicine, it was called the "Persian fire."

Diabetes may lead to many complications, attacking various vital organs. One of its complications is a special kind of nephritis (inflamation of the kidneys). Diabetes also frequently affects the eyesight. It may cause cataracts, eye hemorrhages, spots in the retina, and paralysis of muscles.

Diabetics with terminal stages of kidney disease can now receive kidney transplants and be hopeful that the transplants will function well. This is a report received recently from Dr. John S. Najarian, Chairman of the Department of Surgery at the University of Minnesota Hospitals in Minneapolis.

Persons with juvenile diabetes often die of kidney disease (uremia) in their 30's and 40's, but are generally not considered candidates for kidney transplants because they are

---

Additional material touching on this subject can be found in chapters 52 and 88.

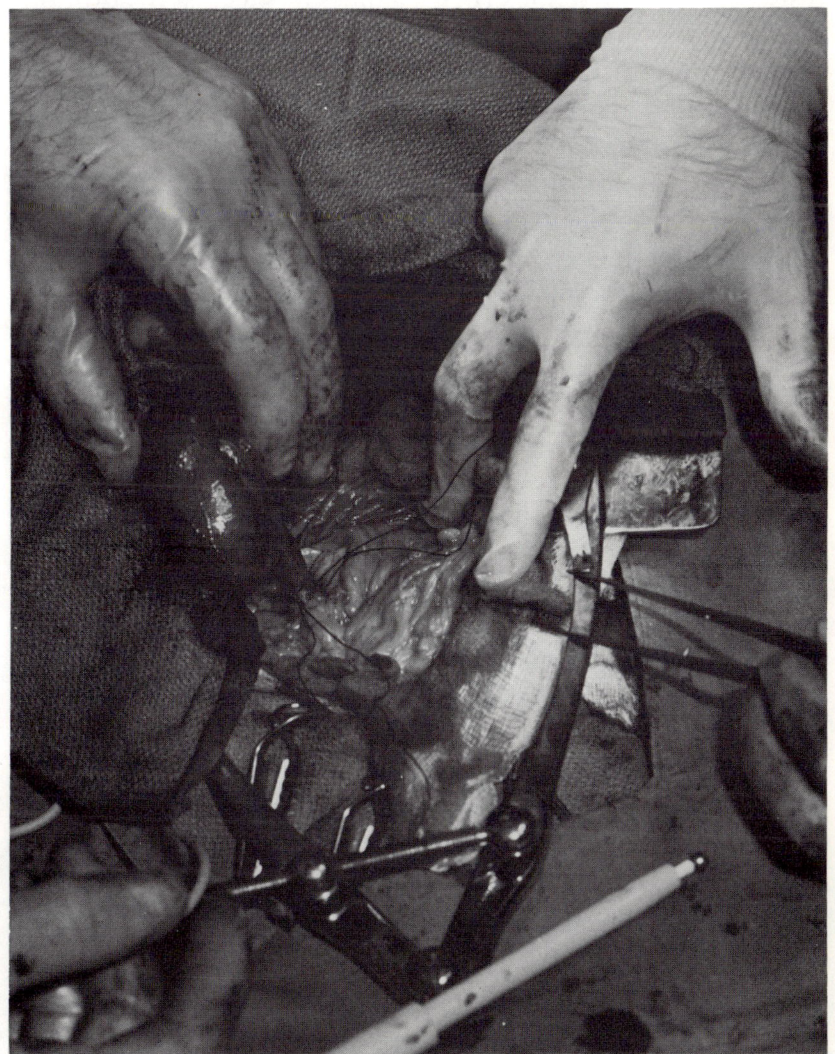

A kidney, being removed, during a kidney transplant operation.

usually poor risks. Doctors feel that diabetes-caused difficulties in wound-healing, steroid tolerance, and infection resistance greatly reduce their chances of success. In addition, the consensus among doctors is that their rehabilitation would be extremely difficult for a number of medical reasons, including the diabetics' propensity for heart disease.

Dr. Najarian does not agree that diabetics should not receive kidney transplants. Thirty-four such transplants have been done at the University since 1966, and about two-thirds of the 31 recipients of transplanted kidneys are still alive. Most have shown improvement in the various diabetes-caused conditions from which they suffer. Bladder control has also been improved in some of the patients.

One of the most impressive effects of the kidney transplant recipients was the stabilization of their eyesight—which remained sharp. Since the loss of vision in these patients was most rapid during the year immediately preceding the transplant, Dr. Najarian suggested that the eyesight of persons suffering from diabetic kidney disease would be better preserved if they receive a transplant kidney before the uremia becomes very severe.

Dr. Najarian's kidney transplant recipients ranged in age from 24 to 55 years, with the largest group being between the ages of 24 and 34. Of the 23 patients who received their kidneys from a related donor, 16 are are now well. Of eight who received the transplant kidneys from cadavers, six are well.

In conclusion, Dr. Najarian feels that diabetics are better candidates for kidney transplants than for hemodialysis and that they should not be absolutely excluded from the benefits of kidney transplants.

55. REVERSING A VASECTOMY

RECENTLY AN estimated one million American men underwent the male sterilization operation known as *vasectomy*. Vasectomy is a relatively simple surgical procedure: The surgeon cuts through the *vas deferens,* the two internal body passages through which the sperm passes on its way toward the penis. Once the vas deferens is cut through, the man is sterile.

Medically, vasectomy is considered an irreversible procedure. Once performed, the operation is final. The severed ends of the vas deferens cannot be re-joined to make the man fertile once more.

Surgeons have attempted to sew back the cut ends of the sperm canals, but these operations have been generally unsuccessful, and even though the cut ends have been joined together, the men have not regained their fertility, for reasons not yet known to doctors. Only about one vasectomy reversal in five succeeds in restoring fertility.

Now, there appears to be some progress in reversing vasectomies. A pioneering vascular surgeon, Dr. Julius H. Jacobson II, of Mt. Sinai Hospital in New York City, has developed a promising new surgical technique which he has used in reversing 20 vasectomies.

Dr. Jacobson's technique involves the use of a microscope

Additional material touching on this subject can be found in chapter 50.

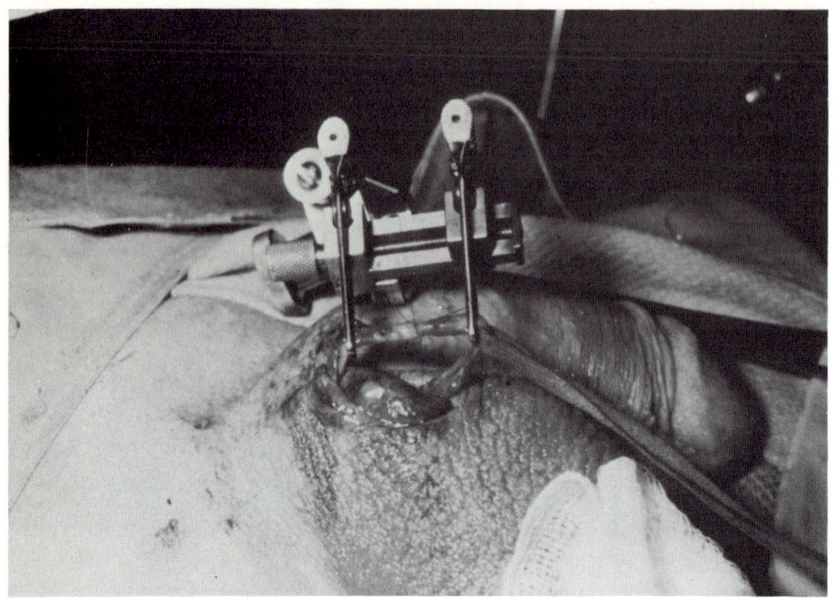

The vas deferens visible as it is being held in an elevated position by a specially devised clamp.

which he developed, and through which the severed ends of each vas stand out sharply, in three dimensions, magnified 25 times their actual size.

Though the sperm canals are fairly large on the outside, they are not hollow tubes. Each sperm tunnel is a tiny slit, about one-fiftieth of an inch across—to the naked eye the openings of the severed ends appear not larger than pinholes. In order to achieve recanalization—restoration of the vas canal—the severed ends must be joined with great precision. If the open ends of the canals do not meet perfectly, the recanalization fails.

Dr. Jacobson, through the use of the microscope, sews the tiny ends together employing microsurgical needles about the shape and size of an eyelash, and silk sutures finer than human hair.

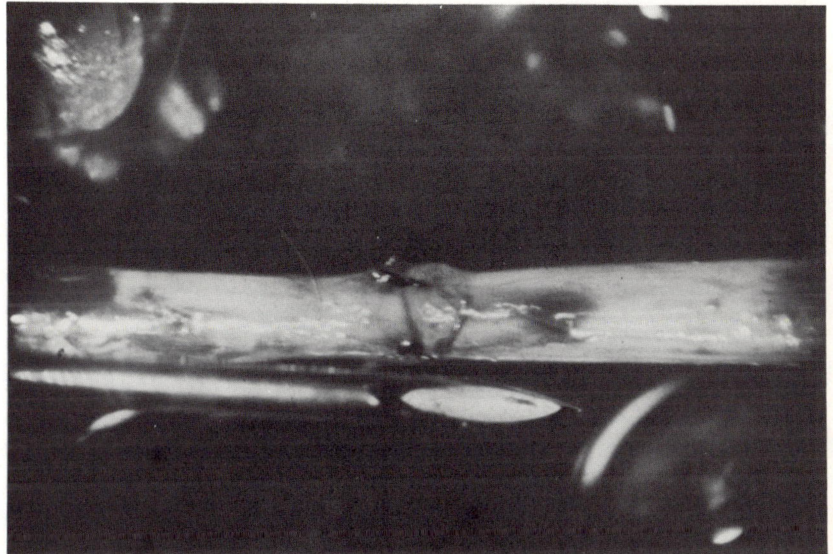

A close-up view of the vas deferens following its repair.

Twenty-five of the 26 men operated on by Dr. Jacobson achieved recanalization—the highest reported rate anywhere in the country—and were able to ejaculate ample quantities of sperm. The wives of four of them became pregnant. As for the others, it is too soon to follow-up, or information is not yet available.

56. THE NEAR-BLIND
CAN SEE AGAIN

PEOPLE WITH CORRECTED VISION of 20/200 (10% of natural vision), or worse, are legally blind in the United States. They are entitled to the blind person's exemption when they file their income tax returns.

About one million people in this country are partially blind and cannot read a newspaper, watch TV, or drive a car with ordinary eyeglasses because they have 10% or less vision.

Now, thanks to an invention called Zoom Glasses, thousands of these people may be able to see—and do—many things they couldn't before.

The glasses are the invention of a New York optometrist, Dr. William Feinbloom, who has previously invented special opera-like glasses worn by doctors to do delicate surgery.

Dr. Feinbloom's glasses increase vision 600% to 1,000%, allowing persons who are nearly blind to see well enough to read a newspaper. Those with as little vision as two percent are able to read again with these glasses, while those with a 10% vision can have their sight improved to a point where they are able—and legally allowed—to drive an automobile.

The Zoom Glasses, which look like miniature telescopes, have two lenses. The front lens is made from plastic, about 14" in diameter; the rear lens is made of glass, about one inch

---

Additional material touching on this subject can be found in chapters 9, 21, 25, 30, 36 and 70.

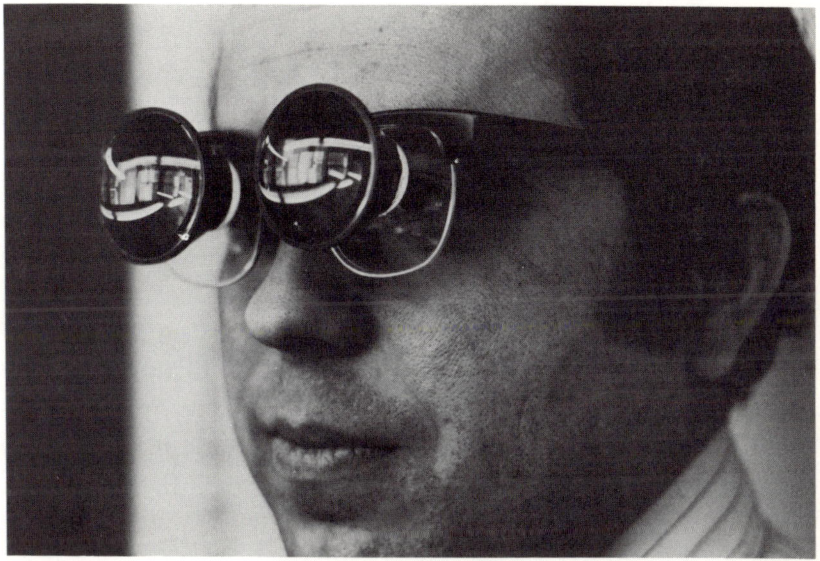

Zoom glasses for the near-blind.

in diameter. The lenses are about an inch apart, and they can be zoomed to the patient's vision requirements and then locked.

Though they look bizarre and heavy, they don't bother the wearer, and they are lighter than they look. They are made an integral part of the patient's eyeglasses. (Most near-blind people wear glasses.) By using hinged sunglass shades, the glasses can be masked by the wearer who feels too conspicuous in them.

The zoom glasses have to be fitted individually for each wearer, and Dr. Feinbloom has instructed many doctors in his technique. The cost of the glasses varies from $600 to $800. Dr. Feinbloom has not patented his magic glasses, because he wants them available to all who need them.

57. ELECTRICITY FOR RELIEF OF INTRACTABLE PAIN

INTRACTABLE PAIN—chronic pain that will not go away and cannot be relieved with drugs—can become so severe as to be totally disabling. Various conditions—diabetes, arthritis, nerve inflammations—cause agonizing, chronic pain, but the most common of them are advanced cancer and chronic backache.

The only relief from intractable pain usually lies in very heavy doses of narcotics—which grow progressively heavier as the patient's body adjusts itself to the drug—that relieve the pain, but also kill the appetite, dull the intellect, and reduce the patient to a living vegetable.

Sometimes, surgery involving severing of the nerves relieves the pain. This, however, always involves major surgery requiring total anesthesia—and it is not always practical. Often, intractable pain comes as an after-effect of major surgery—for example, surgery to remove a cancer tumor—and the patient is too weak to tolerate another round with the knife.

Now, a Florida physician, Dr. Hubert L. Rosomoff, chairman of the Department of Neurological Surgery at the University of Miami School of Medicine, has developed a new technique for relieving intractable pain without surgery.

The new procedure is called a *percutaneous cordotomy,*

---

and since 1964, Dr. Rosomoff has used it to relieve pain in 800 patients. Immediate and complete pain relief has been achieved in 80 percent of the patients, while another 13 percent of the patients no longer have to depend upon drugs for relief.

In the procedure, a hollow needle is inserted into the spinal cord, under local anesthesia. The patient is awake and is able to tell the doctor how the procedure is affecting his pain. The needle is inserted in the spinal cord which contains the nerves causing the pain, and always on the opposite side of the painful area, since nerves controlling pain cross over inside the spinal cord.

The doctor who inserts the needle is guided by a special X-ray TV unit, and once the needle is in place, a thin wire is pushed in through the needle until it touches the correct spot on the spinal cord. This wire is the electrode through which radio frequency current is sent to destroy the nerves. The current is applied in short bursts, with the surgeon watching the patient's reaction to the procedure. The relief is immediate and the patient is free of pain before the procedure is completed.

In some patients, where the pain is on both sides of the body, the procedure has to be done twice, once on each side. In others, it has to be repeated for various reasons, such as the occasional return of pain. This is not dangerous, and the procedure may be repeated any number of times.

Though the percutaneous cordotomy does not involve the use of a knife, it is a serious procedure. The spinal canal and the spinal cord are very small and the area is crowded with vital motor nerves which might be affected or damaged during the procedure if the electrode is even slightly off, which does happen since it's impossible to site it with absolute precision every time. Also, the very nature of entering the spinal cord with a strange object produces side effects. Both the side effects caused by the off-site electrode, and the natural side effects resulting from the entry of the needle, are usually minor and not lasting.

The one permanent after-effect is loss of ability to feel hot or cold in the spot relieved of pain. There is also a possibility of lasting side effects in the performance of sexual functions, but statistics on this have been impossible to gather.

Lastly, there is a possibility of death as a result of this procedure. This can happen if the electrode should come into contact with nerves controlling respiration.

The risks of the operation must be weighed against the benefits. For those with terminal cancer, it may bring welcome relief for the remaining months, or years, since not all terminal cancer patients die soon after contracting the ailment. For those suffering from disabling pain caused by non-lethal diseases, particularly for those who are young and have a lifetime ahead of them—or would, if they had no pain—it may mean a return to a tolerable, normal existence.

58. A CONTRACEPTIVE IMPLANT EFFECTIVE FOR ONE YEAR

THE SEARCH FOR an effective, easy-to-use, safe contraceptive device continues unabated everywhere in the world. The many contraceptive devices available today are all wanting either in complete effectiveness, convenience or safety. Many are troublesome, cumbersome and require a large degree of motivation for their continuous use, which many women do not have.

The "pill" has not solved the problem either. Many women can't take them for health reasons; others can't seem to remember to take them regularly. The best solution appears to be a contraceptive device which could be implanted in the uterus and would require no attention from the wearer for long periods of time. Doctors are now testing such devices which contain *progesterone*.

Progesterone, a hormone which is secreted by the body after ovulation, is a "natural drug" which prevents pregnancy. Progesterone can pass through the walls of silicone rubber capsules at a reasonably constant rate of secretion, preventing a pregnancy when a progesterone-filled capsule is placed in the woman's uterus.

However, two problems have been found to exist when the capsules are actually used in humans. One problem is that the rate of hormone release is not always constant. The second is that the capsule does not always stay where it has been placed.

The first problem appears to have been solved by a team of researchers, led by Dr. Antonio Scommenga of the Michael Reese Hospital, in Chicago. Dr. Scommenga has found that the use of a soft material called silastic (made by Dow Corning) has made it possible to control the release of the hormone into the body by adjusting the concentration of the hormone inside the capsule. Also, Dr. Scommenga's team has determined the exact spot inside the uterus where the capsule is to be placed for best results.

The other problem is that of expulsion of the capsule from the uterus by natural contractions. Dr. Scommenga's team tried various shapes of capsules—triangles, loops, rings, etc—to determine which shape would stay in place the longest, and to find out which shape causes the least number of side effects, such as bleeding and infection, which are common to all IUDs (intra-uterine devices). None of the shapes tested was found to be completely satisfactory. All had a high expulsion rate. However, all that stayed in place worked perfectly to prevent pregnancy. No pregnancy occurred with a progesterone-filled IUD in place.

Dr. Scommenga is continuing his work on the determination of the ideal shape for the hoped-for once-a-year contraceptive. And commercial interest in the new possibility is great. To date, however, no progesterone-filled IUD has been approved by the government for sale to the public.

A Palo Alto, California-based manufacturer, Alza Corporation, received wide publicity when it reported that it intended to seek government approval to market its progesterone-filled IUD. The Alza device is a small T-shaped plastic loop filled with progesterone, designed to be inserted in the uterus where it would secrete minute quantities of the birth control hormone for a period of one year. The company has reported that it tested the device in 2,000 women, only one of whom became pregnant. Alza also reported a very low expulsion rate, but the combined reasons for removal is still fairly high, although lower than any conventional IUD. Alza is continuing to seek government approval for it and if successful, it will become the first on the market.

59. NEW DEVICE PROVIDES ON-THE-SPOT OXYGEN

MANY PERSONS suffering from chronic heart conditions, emphysema or other respiratory ailments rely on an immediate supply of oxygen for emergency or prescribed medical treatment.

Until now there were only two ways to ensure an immediate supply of oxygen. One could duplicate a hospital installation of big steel bottles filled with compressed gas, semipermanently mounted, and exchanged when empty. Or, one carried around a portable steel tank with a limited supply of compressed oxygen—an expensive and often inconvenient and inadequate arrangement.

Now, a portable device is available which makes an emergency supply of oxygen available anywhere, anytime—in the automobile, on a boat or on the golf course. The SOS-Solid Oxygen System delivers from fifteen to forty-five minutes supply of 99.9 percent pure oxygen from a lightweight (4.4 pounds) set of canisters in a stylish case with a shoulder strap.

The secret is in the form of the oxygen. It comes in *solid* form, encased in metal canisters the size of small juice concentrate cans. Each 12-ounce canister produces 15 minutes worth of pure moisturized oxygen. The canister holds solid material (a cake of sodium chlorate mixed with a catalyst) which is converted to oxygen at the push of a button. The button drives a needle inside the top of the canister through a

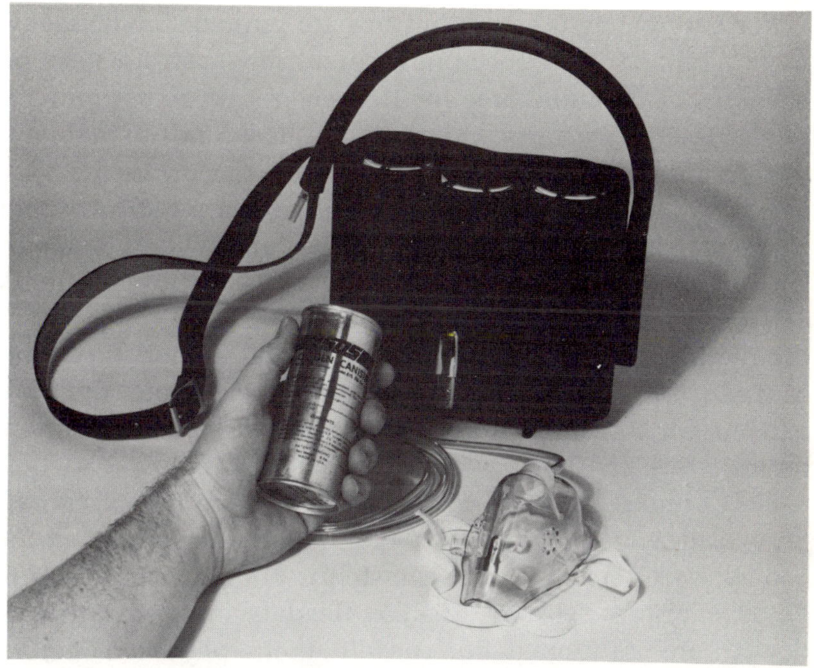

The SOS (Solid Oxygen System) mask, replacement canisters and carrying case. Insertion of the canisters into the dispenser requires only seconds. With the latch released and the dispenser in an upside down position, three canisters are inserted into wire supports (visible above).

capsule of water, allowing the water to seep down through the solid material inside, causing a chemical reaction which produces gaseous oxygen and a small amount of water. There are no confusing dials, gauges, valves or regulators, and the pressure produced in the canister is so low that danger of explosion—always present with gaseous or liquid oxygen dispensers—is eliminated.

The canisters fit into a 3-canister dispenser that weighs two pounds and has the attractive appearance of a binocular case with a suede-like finish. Oxygen from the canisters passes through a clear, plastic tube in the carrying strap to a soft, clear face mask. Each canister provides a minimum of 4 liters of oxygen per minute for 15 minutes.

For emergency use, two buttons are pushed simultaneously, providing 8 liters per minute, or all three canisters can be activated at the same time for 12 liters of oxygen per minute. Replacement canisters can be inserted in seconds to maintain the required required availability of oxygen as long as necessary. Full canisters are marked with a pink dot which changes to blue when used. The outlet tube is equipped with an oxygen flow indicator which shows when the canister is empty.

the required availability of oxygen as long as necessary. Full canisters are marked with a pink dot which changes to blue when used. The outlet tube is equipped with an oxygen flow indicator which shows when the canister is empty.

This unique system is made by Life Support, Inc., 907 E. Strawbridge Ave., Melbourne, Florida. The dispenser sells for $98.50; a six-pack of oxygen canisters is $14.95; an econo-pack of 30 canisters sells for $64.95. Readers interested in this device are cautioned to consult their physician before purchasing it.

60. TAMING A RARE TIC WITH TRANQUILIZER

EVERYONE BLINKS. But when blinking persists it might be Gilles de la Tourette's disease—a rare disorder, often poorly understood and misdiagnosed by physicians. It is named after the Frenchman who first described it back in 1825. Until now, no effective treatment for it was known.

Tourette's disease occurs between the ages of two and 14 years. It often starts as mere eye blinks. Parents, teachers and physicians tend to believe that the symptoms of the disease, especially the early ones, are habits or common tics of childhood which will disappear. When the symptoms persist, they are often thought to be of a psychological nature.

Tourette's disease is a maze of symptoms which change, and disappear, but then return. It generally starts with a tic-like movement—usually; at first, a simple facial tic. With time, new tics develop and replace, or are added to, old ones. The tics are rhythmical, purposeless and rapid—from one to 1,000 tics per hour. They are always involuntary.

Involuntary noises, described as barks, grunts and hisses are also common initial symptoms. Movements usually progress from simple to complicated, giving the appearance of being purposeful, but, in fact, are entirely involuntary. Even though the person afflicted with the disease is fully aware of his condition and may try to suppress it, he cannot do so.

Involuntary noises—sounds or words—eventually appear

in all persons afflicted with the illness, but its most famous symptom—*coprolalia*—appears in only about half of the cases. Coprolalia is the involuntary repetition of vulgar or obscene words. A person afflicted with it constantly repeats obscene words and epithets with full realization of what he is doing, yet unable to stop it. What is most interesting is that despite common belief that these people are crazy, there is no mental deterioration at all. The cause of the disease is unknown.

The disease has—or can develop—many other symptoms, including repetitive touching and *echolalia*—repeating what someone else has said. It is a very unpleasant affliction and becomes progressively worse with age. Life becomes a tragedy for the afflicted person.

Effective treatment of the disease is now possible with the tranquilizer *haloperidol*, according to psychiatrist Dr. Arthur K. Shapiro, director of the Special Studies Laboratory at the Payne Whitney Psychiatric Clinic of New York Hospital-Cornell Medical Center in Manhattan.

Basing his claim on the study of the largest group of Tourette's disease victims in the country, Dr. Shapiro says that four out of five patients treated with haloperidol obtain a 95-99 percent cure, and the fifth gets about 80 percent relief. The treatment with the tranquilizer may take as long as a year before the proper dose is determined.

Dr. Shapiro favors starting with high, powerful doses of the drug, reducing the dosage as the symptoms decrease. The drug causes some severe and unpleasant side effects, and treatment must be carefully regulated to balance the relief from the symptoms and the ability to tolerate side effects. Once the balance is achieved, the patient can be maintained on very low doses of the tranquilizer.

61. REANIMATING PARALYZED SPHINCTERS

SINCE 1968, Dr. Noel Thompson, of the Middlesex Hospital in London has used muscle transplants, in an effort to improve functions in 40 patients with unilateral (one-sided) facial palsy, and seven others with cleft palate and inadequate speech.

Facial palsy (paralysis) can happen as a result of a disease, such as geniculate herpes (a disease of the facial nerve) or Bell's palsy (a paralysis of the sides of the face, often affecting the eyelids), or it may be congenital. Facial paralysis also occurs as the after-effect of various surgical procedures, such as mastoidectomy, parotidectomy or craniotomy. Breaking the base of the skull in an accident can also paralyze various facial muscles.

The circular muscles which control the functions of body openings, such as the anus, the mouth and the eyes are called sphincters. These are the muscles which must be reconstructed in order to relieve the paralysis. Muscle transplants were first tried over 100 years ago, but have commonly failed over the years because the muscle proved unable to survive the denial of oxygen for more than a few hours. Since it required some time for the transplanted muscle to "take" in its new location, and to receive a regular supply of oxygen from the blood, it could not survive.

Dr. Thompson found that the secret of muscle survival in

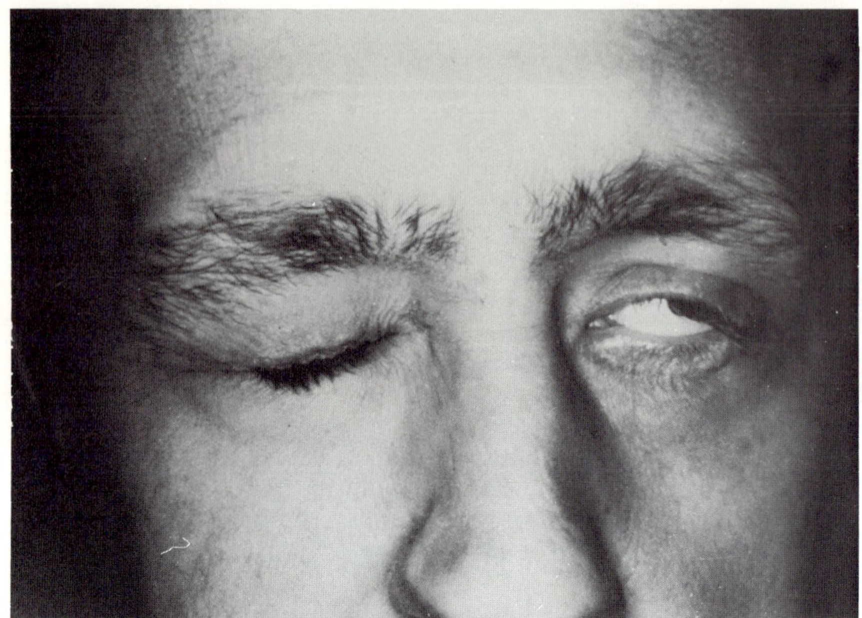

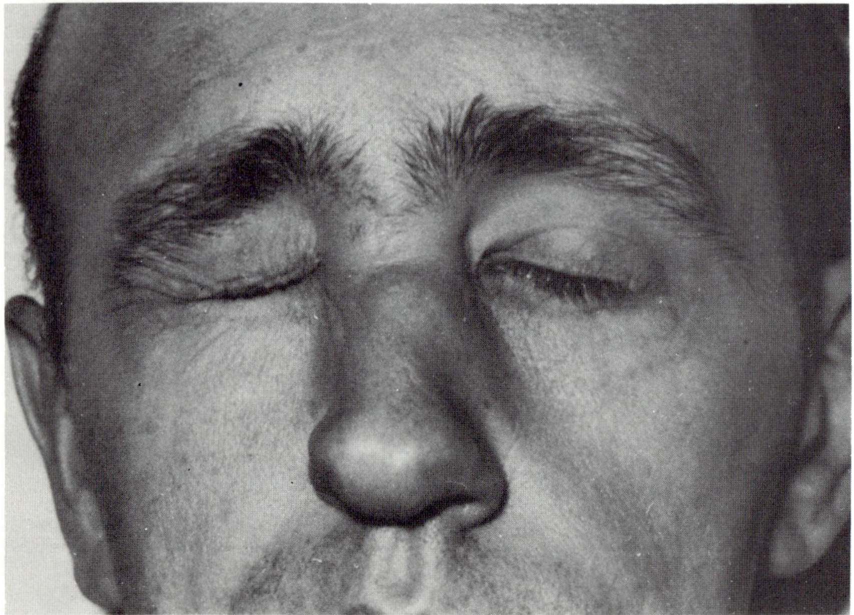

The patient pictured, age 39, had complete facial paralysis before the muscle transplant (top) which prevented him from closing his eyelids properly. The bottom photo shows the improved condition one year after the transplant.

transplants is in reducing its need for oxygen. This he accomplishes by denervation of the muscle selected for the transplant two weeks before the actual operation.

Denervation is done by cutting off the nerve supply to the muscle, without removing the muscle itself. Dr. Thompson starts the transplant procedure when he denervates a muscle in the forearm or in the foot, by incisions which cut off its nerve supply. Then, two or three weeks later, he removes the muscle and immediately transplants it to its new location.

The results of the transplants have been excellent. Out of 28 reconstructions of the oral (mouth) sphincter, only one graft failed to "take." In the others, normal mouth function was restored in 82% of the patients, and the other 14% were markedly improved. The repair of the eye muscles, to restore function to paralyzed eyelids, produced good to satisfactory results in 19 out of 20 patients.

The muscles taken from the forearm or the foot to be used in the operation are "dispensable"—sort of "spares" provided by nature. Their removal has no effect on the arm or on the foot.

An interesting application of muscle transplants is seen in cases of partial facial paralysis, where weakness of elevation in the angle of the mouth may be corrected by grafting new muscle to the weakened face muscle, restoring normal movement.

In cases of cleft palate, muscle transplants have been done by Dr. Thompson to restore normal or acceptable speech in cases where surgical repair has failed to accomplish it. This is done by transplanting the muscle to the palato-pharyngeal sphincter (the muscle which controls the escape of air through the nose).

Dr. Thompson's work promises hope in the reconstruction of the anal and bladder sphincters. This would give new life to many who suffer from paralysis of those vital muscles.

62. REBUILDING
THE HUMAN FACE

A FRENCH PLASTIC surgeon's bold, new technique has resulted in providing "new" faces for some 300 deformed children and adults on whom he operated over the past dozen years.

The surgeon, Dr. Paul Tessier, chief of plastic surgery at the Hospital Foch in Paris, has even made a tour of the United States demonstratng his technique for American doctors.

Dr. Tessier specializes in rebuilding deformed faces caused by various congenital diseases. A number of children are born with rare diseases which deform the face. Often, as the child grows older, the deformities become progressively worse. When the child becomes an adult the condition is evidenced by protruding eyeballs, ulcers in the eyes, double vision, blindness, and difficulties in breathing. The afflicted become hideous individuals, with twisted, grotesque faces.

Though surgeons do not hesitate to rebuild human faces smashed in an accident, many balk at remaking congenital defects. Dr. Tessier's technique is to apply the same principles used in rebuilding a human face damaged in an accident to repairs of congenital deformities. For example, if a man had broken his skull in a car accident, a surgeon would be able to reconstruct it by following established surgical procedures. In

Additional material touching on this subject can be found in chapters 3, 19, 63 and 72.

170

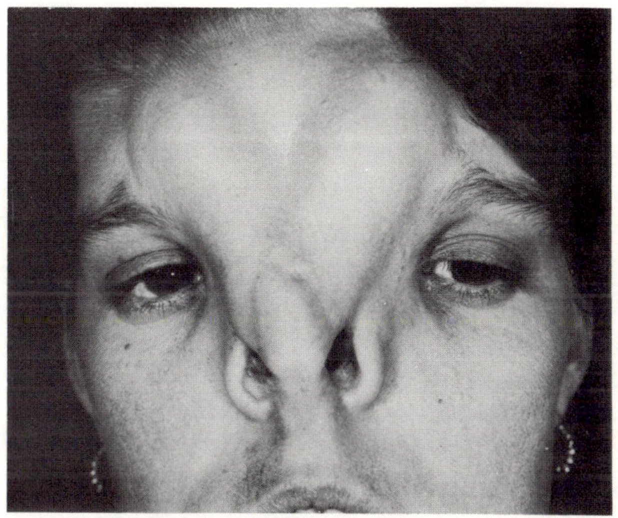

The frontal view of the face of an adult suffering from hypertolism, giant frontal pneumatisation and double alar cleft.

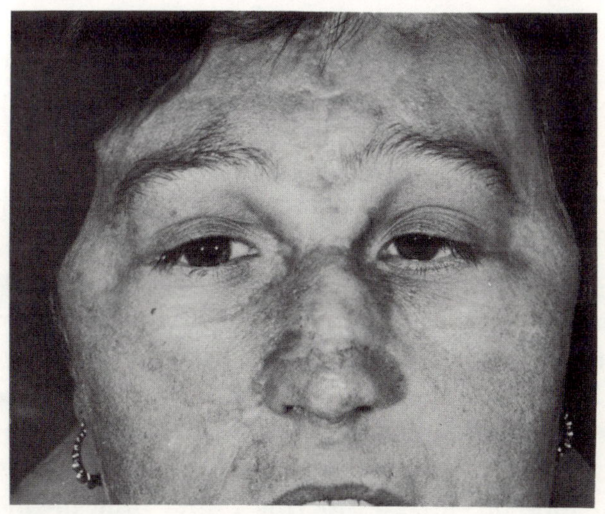

The same person after corrective surgery.

repairing a congenital deformity, Dr. Tessier "breaks" the skull and then goes on to the task of reconstruction as if the patient were in an accident.

The "breaking" of the bones in the face or skull is, of course, surgical cutting. Dr. Tessier calls this procedure, making "controlled" fractures in strategic sites. Before operating, he takes a great many X-rays and, in the case of children, makes a careful analysis of the growth changes that are still developing in the growing face. If he thinks that surgery can correct the defect, he plans a procedure that is individually designed for each patient.

The operations are bold and complex. No procedure is taken lightly or as a matter-of-fact. The various operations involve resecting (removing) large pieces of bones and resetting the bones in new positions. This is accomplished with the help of bone grafts made of bone wedges taken from the patient's ribs, or other dispensible bones. Sometimes, an entire section of the face must be moved inwards or outwards.

For example, to correct hypertolism—abnormally wide separation of the eyes—almost the entire skull must be cut apart and a large chunk of the bone removed from the forehead in order to bring the eye sockets closer together. Not only is this extremely complex surgery, but it requires great skill and experience since the moving of the bones affects the functioning of muscles and nerves, and these facts must be carefully considered. Again, in moving the eye sockets, great care must be taken that the move is sufficiently precise to avoid double vision (a common condition with hypertolism) and yet not to stretch the optic nerve.

Though similar surgery has been attempted in this country, none has been as complex as Dr. Tessier's. After watching Dr. Tessier operate during his visit to the United States, some American surgeons are considering duplicating his methods.

63. TOE CONVERTED INTO THUMB TO RESTORE HAND FUNCTION

SURGEONS AT THE University of California in San Francisco have created a new thumb for a patient by sucessfully transplanting his big toe to his hand.

The medical team of four surgeons was headed by Dr. Harry J. Buncke, Jr., a clinical instructor in plastic surgery who has been studying toe to thumb transplants in monkeys.

Six months after the surgery the new thumb was almost normal in appearance and function, though slightly shorter and wider than a normal thumb. The patient's handwriting has not changed and he reports that the absence of the great toe has not stopped him from water skiing, hiking or climbing ladders. Although he lost his thumb when he accidentally cut it off with a power saw, after the transplant he went back to using power and hand tools. His right hand, with its new thumb, has 80% the grip strength of his uninjured left hand.

The toe to thumb transplant was a voluntary decision of the patient. He wanted to try it in preference to other reconstruction procedures, such as peg prosthesis or bone grafts.

The operation involved was a double one. One team of surgeons prepared the hand, freeing the arteries, tendons and nerves from the scar tissue on the stump of the old thumb. The second team of surgeons removed the big toe, flushed it out and bored a hole into the toe bone.

Additional material touching on this subject can be found in chapters 3, 19, 62 and 72.

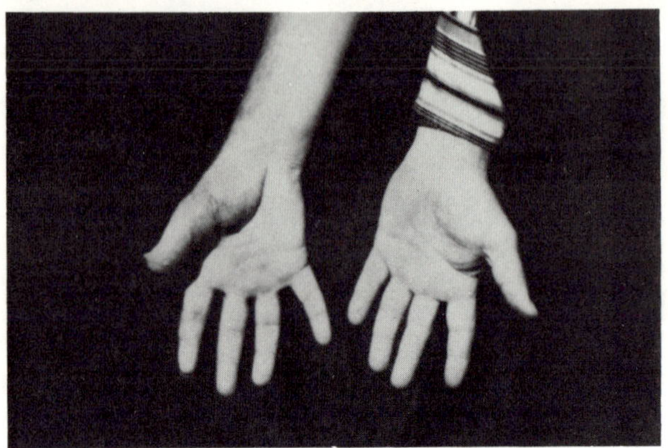

A hand with a toe-thumb (left) compared with a normal hand.

The toe was affixed to the stump bone with a bone peg taken from the patient's right tibia.. The veins, nerves and tendons were stitched together, using a microscope during surgery. Then, the newly transplanted toe was sutured to the skin at the thumb base. The defect on the foot was covered with skin flaps and skin graft.

During the first two days after the transplant surgery the patient had problems. Twice, the artery developed a blood clot and had to be opened to have the clot removed. In addition, there was continuous bleeding the first day, which required a blood transfusion. However, after the second blood clot was removed, the toe/thumb started to improve in color and temperature and there were no further problems. The patient left the hospital sixteen days after the transplant.

The new technique is a promising development for anyone who has lost a thumb. The function of the thumb is of great importance since the hand depends on it to do the work for which it was designed. The big toe is also important, but not nearly as vital as the thumb; and exchanging a big toe for a new thumb might be worth considering.

64. TRANQUILIZER RELIEF FOR ANGINA SUFFERERS

TO ITS THOUSANDS of victims, angina pectoris is more than just a medical name for a heart illness. It's an agonizing, weakening sickness that seldom leaves the individual free of pain for more than a day at a time, and it can turn even the smallest effort—getting into a car, for example—into an ordeal. An attack of angina pectoris means a severe constricting pain in the chest, radiating from the region of the heart to the left shoulder and down the arm. It is sometimes accompanied by apprehension of immediate death.

In recent years, medical studies have pointed out that there is psychosomatic basis for some forms of heart disease. These studies show that mental strain is a possible factor in arteriosclerotic heart disease.

A small-scale study conducted by Dr. Marvin L. Bierenbaum, director of the Atherosclerosis Research Group at the St. Vincent's Hospital in Montclair, New Jersey, suggests that the calming properties of tranquilizers may relieve some victims of angina pectoris.

The study used a tranquilizer called diazepam—better known under its "drug store name" of Valium—but Dr. Bierenbaum says he can make a "philosophical guess" that

---

Additional material touching on this subject can be found in chapters 7, 24, 32, 84, 94, 96, 98 and 99.

other tranquilizers might also be effective in lessening the frequency and severity of angina attacks.

Ten married men, ages 48 to 60 years, participated in the test study. All had arteriosclerotic heart disease and angina pectoris. They came in every other week, for a total of three sessions. At the first session, the men were examined, had blood samples taken, and were given the medicine to take at home. Some were given diazepam, others a placebo—a "make-believe" pill which looked like the real thing but contained no drugs. None of the men knew what he was taking during the study. At the next session, the pills were switched, so that each man had been studied for effects both ways—with the drug, and without it (using only the placebo).

To subject the men to mental stress each was given a mirror drawing test. In this test, patients trace a star reflected in a mirror. The test is not easy. "It's quite frustrating unless you have tremendous dexterity or ability," says Dr. Bierenbaum. To add to the stress, each patient was told: The other fellows did a little better."

Tests of blood samples taken after the sessions showed a reduced anxiety in six of the nine men (one dropped out of the study) and all six reported a decrease in the frequency and severity of their angina attacks. Three men did not respond to the stress test. These three continued in a highly anxious state and had much less angina relief from the tranquilizer. It is probable that they needed larger doses of diazepam.

65. A MEDICINE FOR MALIGNANT OTITIS

MALIGNANT EXTERNAL OTITIS is a severe infection which originates in the outer ear. It usually attacks elderly diabetics. It begins insidiously, accompanied by progressive pain and a discharge of pus from the ear. It sometimes starts following a minor injury to the ear.

The infection spreads inside the head where it causes *osteomyelitis* (inflammation of the bone marrow) of the temporal bone and the base of the skull, facial nerve paralysis, paralysis of cranial nerves, meningitis, brain abscess and death.

Until recently, the chances of survival were poor. The spread of the infection was difficult to stop with surgery, and the organism causing the infection, *pseudomonas aeruginosa*, was resistant to usual antibiotics.

About six years ago a new treatment for malignant external otitis was begun by Dr. J. Ryan Chandler (who gave the disease its name), now Chairman of the Department of Otolaryngology at the University of Miami School of Medicine. It involved a combination of surgery and an antibiotic drug called *gentamicin*, not generally used until now for treatment of this infection. In 1970, Dr. Chandler started to treat malignant otitis with a new drug, *disodium carbenicillin*, and he has found that the infection can be treated in a conservative fashion. Of his last 15 patients, 13 were treated with *carbenicillin* and *gentamicin*. Only six required surgery and only one died.

Since he started the new treatments, in 1968, Dr. Chandler has treated 38 patients having an average age of 71. Thirty-six of them were diabetics. The treatments started at various stages of the disease. Sixteen of the patients were in the stage of facial paralysis, and Dr. Chandler was able to save eight of them. Early treatment is recommended, says Dr. Chandler, because once the facial paralysis sets in it is a sign that the infection has spread deeply inside and chances of survival are dim.

The treatment Dr. Chandler now recommends starts with the debridement of the ear canal (surgical cleaning out). Then, the cavity is packed daily with wicks impregnated with gentamicin ointment. Patients are hospitalized and given injections of gentamicin and carbenicillin almost every hour, around the clock. Pain generally disappears within 36 to 48 hours. Tenderness takes longer to disappear. If the pain persists or the infection spreads, Dr. Chandler operates and makes a wide local incision, which he packs with gauze impregnated with gentamicin ointment.

The nature of malignant external otitis and its manner of insidious attack on the body, point out the importance of promptly seeing a physician whenever a person suffers from continuous earache or whenever there is any discharge from the ear.

66. NEW VEHICLE
FOR THE HANDICAPPED

A WEST GERMAN engineer, Heinz Weinert of Cologne, developed a vehicle for handicapped children and adults which is considered a small revolution in the field of medical-aid vehicles.

Mr. Weinert's motivation in wanting to make life easier for the handicapped was very strong: his daughter Claudia is a thalidomide child, born without normal arms. Mr. Weinert spent three years on the construction of the first "electromobile" and is now making improved models.

The Koelner Elektromobil, as the vehicle is called, is a motorized wheel chair suitable for persons without arms or legs, or for paralytics. The seat is raised or lowered by pushing a button. It is cushioned and upholstered in soft leather which conforms to the shape of the body, thus preventing the formation of any pressure sores. When the seat is lowered all the way down to "floor" level, foot supports slide out from the body of the chair. The buttons controlling the operations of the chair can be pushed with the chin, if necessary.

For use in a room, the distance from the front to the rear axles (the length of the chair) is the same as in a conventional wheel chair. For street use, the push of a button stretches the chair out, increasing the axle's distance by almost a foot. The added length makes for a smoother ride and prevents the elec-

Additional material touching on this subject can be found in chapters 8 and 37.

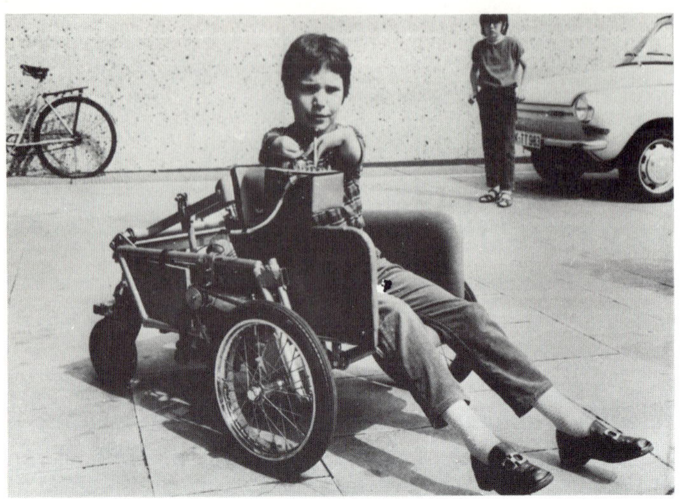

Heinz Weinert's daughter, Claudia, demonstrating the
first electromobile built by her father.

tromobil from tipping over.

The weight of the person using the vehicle is not important
as it is automatically compensated for by pneumatic springs.
Through a simple procedure of changing some of the screws,
the inner configuration of the unit can be adjusted from child-
size to adult-size, and an appropriate size seat is easily installed making it possible for the elektromobil to "grow" with
the child.

Propulsion of the unit is regulated by an electronic drive
unit which permits gentle, slow starts, and gradual changes of
speed. Because of the equalization of weight units and the
electronic drive, only a small electric motor is necessary to
move the vehicle. A sidewalk-climbing attachment is now being tested and if it turns out to be satisfactory, it will be
available for future installation in the vehicles.

The Koelner Elektromobil is now in production on on-order
basis at Ingenieurbuero Weinert, Subblerather Strasse, 5,
Koeln 30, West Germany. The price of an electromobile,
which is hand-made, is presently around $2,000.

67. TUNE IN AND
TUNE OUT HEADACHES

A TEAM OF research workers at the Hadassah-Hebrew University Medical Center in Israel has developed a small machine, the size of a transistor radio, which induces somnolence, tranquility and relaxation in many persons suffering from insomnia, hypertension, allergic asthma, headaches and certain types of migraine.

The "Tranquility Machine," as it is called, was developed by J. Tannenbaum of the Hadassah Electronic Department. It is a transistorized electrical box, (5½" x 5½" x 2½") which is a source of low intensity electrical current, and can be used at home. There is a built-in time switch, which permits the patient to set it for any specific length of time.

In the case of headaches, the patient places three electrodes on his head as near as possible to the painful area. He then sets the timer and relaxes. The electrical stimulation induced by the machine apparently works on the higher centers of the brain—those connected with pain or emotion. A state of somnolence and relaxation bordering on sleep results which, in many cases, relieves symptoms of pain and tension.

In recent years, the Electro-Sleep Clinic at the Hadassah-Hebrew University Medical Center has also functioned as a headache clinic. The main purpose of the clinic is to study the

---

Additional material touching on this subject can be found in chapters 48, 57, 79, 85 and 91.

effect of electrical current treatment in three different types of headaches—tension headache, migraine and post-traumatic headache.

The patients are referred to the clinic by the hospital neurologist. Here they undergo *electroencephalography* (EEG), X-ray of the head and cervical spine, *electromyography* of the neck muscles, and a number of psychological tests. This is done under the supervision of a team consisting of Dr. Florella Magora, the head of the clinic, and a neurologist, psychologist, and physical medicine specialist.

When the machine is switched on, a pleasant sensation is felt all over the head—almost like a hand massage. According to Dr. Magora, "not everybody responds to this gentle electrical stimulation by the machine. But we have now had more than five years of experience with patients using our machine. It is very easy to find out who will respond and who will not. A large number of our patients come to us because they have headaches which no drugs seem able to help.

"We have, for instance, a lawyer who comes when he simply cannot work in his office because his head aches so badly. After using the machine for one hour, he is refreshed and ready to return to work.

"One thing we are sure about after our five years' experience with the machine: There are no side-effects which are harmful to the patient."

Dr. Magora continues: "We believe that after the preliminary investigations have been made by the physician, the patient who has been shown to respond to the machine can quite safely use the machine in his own home. All he has to do is to sit comfortably, perhaps in the living room in front of the television, place the electrodes in position, switch on the time clock, and he will reach a state of relaxed somnolence. When he awakes, in many cases he will have lost his headache, or in the case of insomnia, have had a good night's

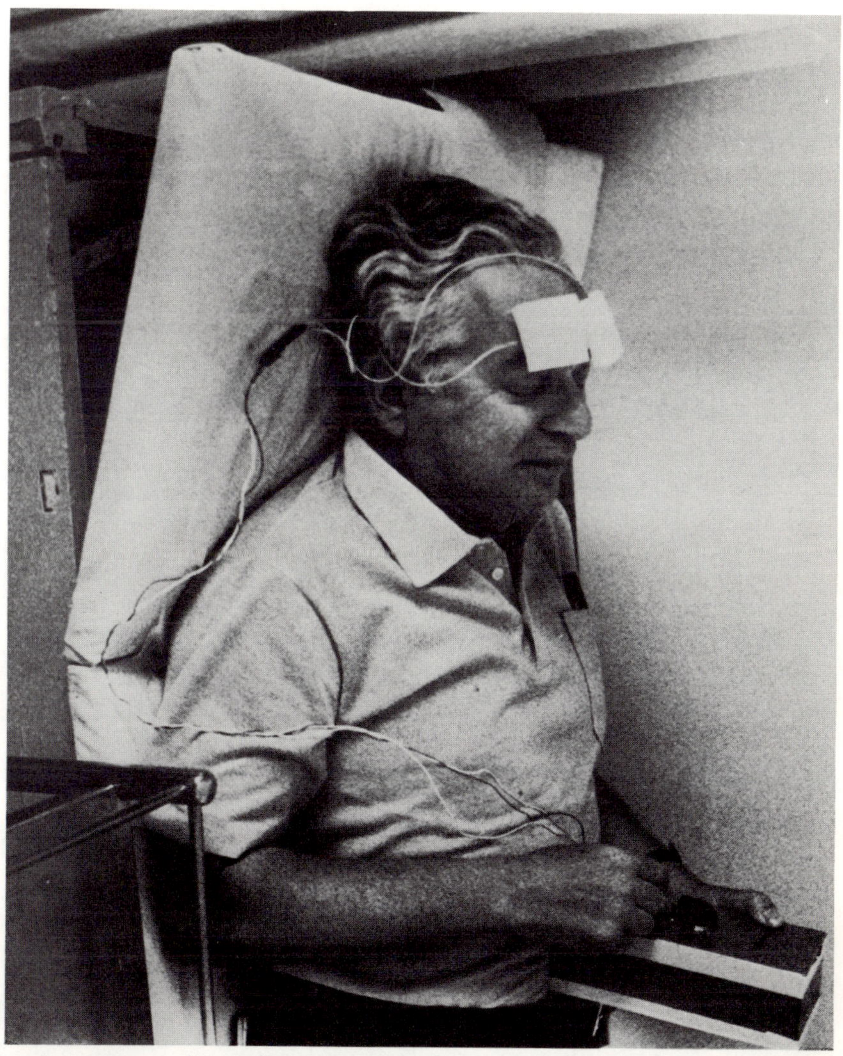

A patient at the Hadassah Hebrew University Hospital tuning out his headache with a Tranquility Machine.

rest and be ready for work. There is no wasting of time in hospital clinics."

The tranquility machine is now being readied for commercial production. At the moment, several of these units, made in the medical center's own workshops, are being used in their outpatient department.

68. CHRONIC RHINITIS RELIEVED WITH CRYOTHERAPY

CHRONIC RHINITIS is an inflammation of the nasal membrane, usually accompanied by a copious discharge. In the later stages, there is a thickening of the membrane and the glands. Treatment includes oral decongestants, silver nitrate-cautery, "painting" with phenol, electrocautery and surgical resection.

Now, cryosurgery has been shown to be more satisfactory than conventional treatment. The results of the new technique were reported by Dr. James M. Ozenberger, professor of otolaryngology at Yale University School of Medicine, who has used it on 145 patients.

Dr. Ozenberger has found that there is always an improvement in the nasal obstruction—ranging from improved to complete—and most patients also reported a reduced discharge. Even patients who were not aware of any nasal obstruction have reported an improvement in the nasal airway. In one group of 46 patients, 72% had complete relief from nasal obstruction and 32% had complete relief from the discharge.

The procedure is carried out by inserting a cryoprobe through the nose and applying freon to the diseased tissue—freezing it. The doctor can watch the position of the cryoprobe with a dental mirror inserted through the mouth.

Additional material touching on this subject can be found in chapters 16 and 38.

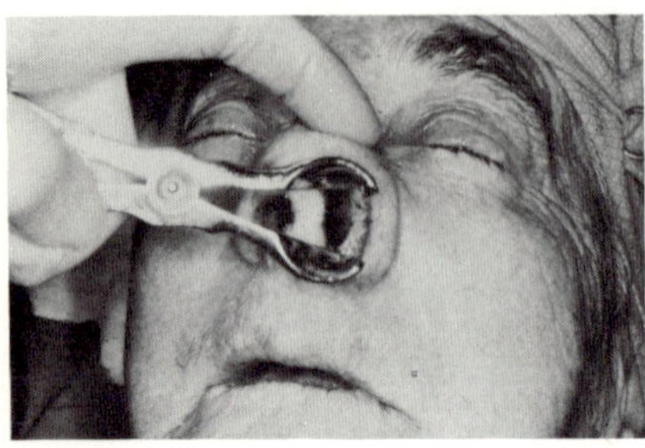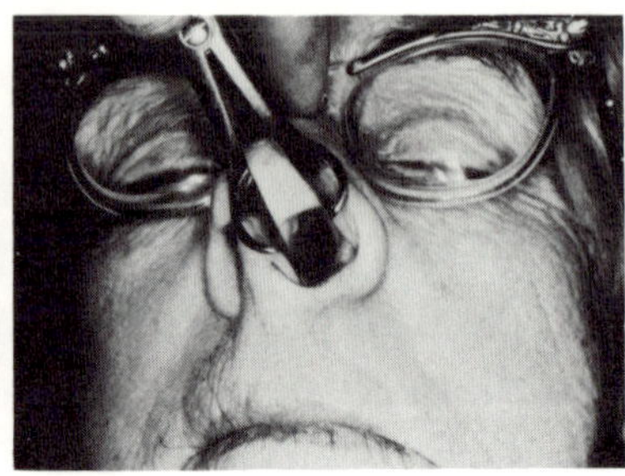

A patient with nasal obstruction (left) and the same patient three years later with a very good airway.

The surgery is done under local anesthesia and does not require any hospitalization—it can be performed in the doctor's office.

A few days after the freezing, the patient returns for removal of the frozen tissue. Some of the patients have to make a second visit to the doctor to remove crusts which have formed during the healing, while others are able to clear the debris themselves.

Dr. Ozenberger has also used cryosurgery with good results to treat nasal tumors, to stop bleeding after a biopsy in patients with small, benign tumors, to treat patients with allergies—and resulting polyps—and to treat patients with epistaxis (nosebleed).

69. DEVELOPING SEXUAL MUSCLES THROUGH EXERCISE

AN ANCIENT EXERCISE to develop sexual muscles in the woman's vagina is now being used in sexual therapy. The purpose is to heighten sexual adequacy, create vaginal awareness, and increase the possibility of orgasm, which might otherwise be impossible.

The idea of using the P.C. to enhance sexual performance is centuries old. A 16th century Hindu book of sexual instructions advised the female to learn to "close and contract the vagina until she holds the penis as with a finger, opening and shutting at her pleasure, and finally acting as the hand of the girl who milks the cow." This ancient practice is now being advised in various gynecological centers, as part of the total picture of sexual therapy, though it is not considered a "magic cure" for nonorgasmic women. However, counselors at the American Institute of Family Relations have taught nonorgasmic women to use their new vagina-contracting ability in intercourse, and obtained good results.

The exercise has been used by gynecologists for years, to restore the function of vaginal muscles after childbirth, after vaginal operations, and also in order to treat poor urine control. However, only recently have doctors come to realize that the exercise has value in sexual therapy.

The technique involves training the woman to tighten and

contract her vaginal muscle which is called the *pubococcygeus,* or P.C. Some women have naturally developed vaginal muscles—to the point of being able to pick up coins with the vagina—but the majority have not developed their sexual muscles, and often are not even aware they exist. Studies conducted by Dr. Arnold H. Kegel, a California gynecologist, show that in at least two out of three women the P.C. is weak and as a consequence, sexual satisfaction minimal.

Actual training in the processes of strengthening vaginal muscles starts with the woman trying to stop the flow while urinating in sitting position, with knees spread wide apart. Often, this effort automatically contracts the P.C. Once the woman learns to recognize this sensation, she can practice the contractions anytime, anywhere, using contractions during urination to check on her progress. Once she achieves good control she can release a little urine at a time.

Normally, the training starts with 10 contractions in a row, six times daily. Gradually, the contractions are increased to 200-300 daily, spaced out and performed whenever convenient. The exercise takes very little time—squeeze, open; squeeze, open—each taking a fraction of a second. It can be performed anywhere—waiting for the elevator, standing in line at the bank or waiting to be checked out in a grocery store. It takes about six weeks to reach 300 contractions daily, but some women require up to 10 weeks to achieve the goal. Once 200-a-day is reached, further exercise is usually unnecessary. The P.C., now, under normal conditions, remains partially contracted, ready to be tightened at will.

70. A LASER CANE
FOR THE BLIND

A CANE FOR THE BLIND, fitted with a *laser beam obstacle detector*, has been developed and is now being tested by the Veterans Administration.

The laser cane is an adaptation of the conventional long cane and is intended to add environment-probing ability to the conventional unit.

The laser cane probes the environment with three laser beams. These intense beams of light detect dropoffs, straight-ahead obstacles, and obstacles ahead that are situated between chest and head height, warning the traveler with sound and touch signals. The new cane thus provides three important pieces of information not otherwise available to the blind traveler, reducing his tension and making his progress more graceful.

Because the canes are designed for the user of conventional canes, they are not too difficult to adapt to. New users would combine the training required for long cane travel with the instructions for laser beam control.

The three laser "eyes" are fitted in the upper part of the cane, pointed downward, straight ahead and upward. Each sends out a pencil-thin laser beam which spreads out to only one inch at a distance of 10 feet. This makes it possible to

---

Additional material touching on this subject can be found in chapters 9, 21, 25, 30, 36, 56 and 70.

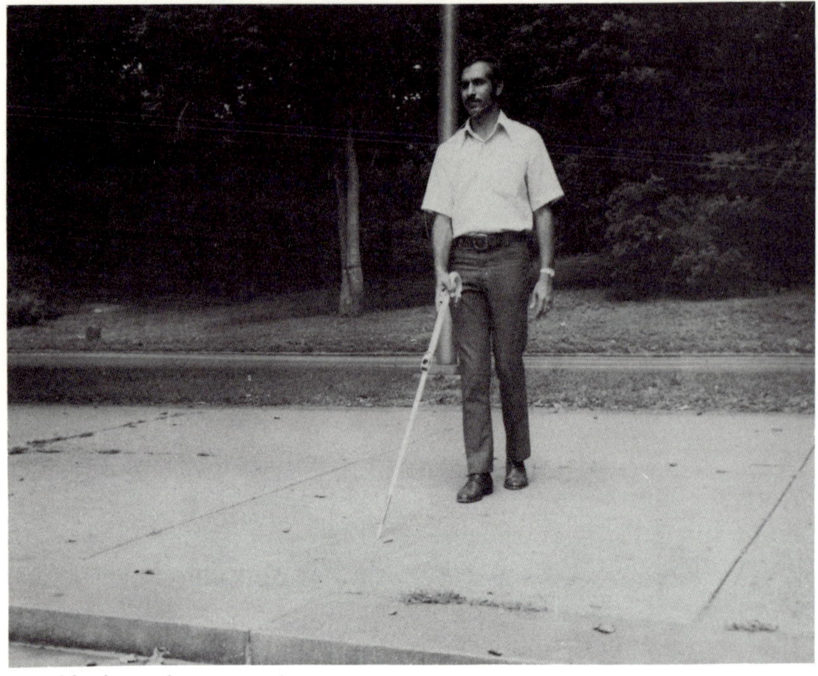

A blind traveler using a laser cane. The mechanical part of the unit can be seen in the upper half of the cane.

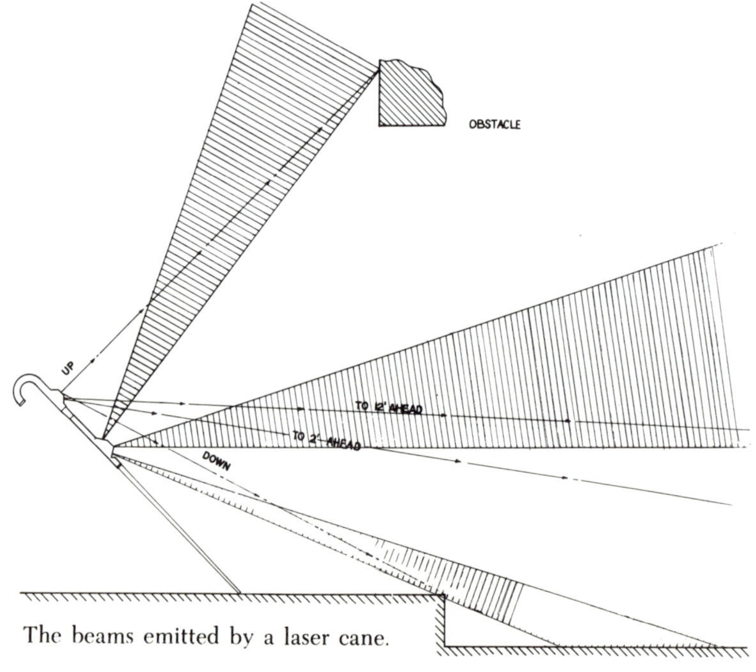

The beams emitted by a laser cane.

locate objects with considerable precision by suitable "fine" scanning. Normal "course" scanning procedure is to sweep the cane back and forth in an arc, using a modified long cane technique.

The cane's downward laser beam warns the traveler, through sound, of any dropoff larger than six inches which is approximately two paces in front of him. Some of the most hazardous dropoffs would be flights of stairs, edges of train platforms, open manholes, and celler-ways.

The straight-ahead beam, about two feet above the ground, can reach out to a maximum distance of 12 feet. The distance is set by a lever located near the user's thumb. Any obstacle detected by the beam activates a touch signal which is felt by the index finger. In addition, a buzzer signal can also be switched on.

The upward-looking beam detects obstacles at head height appearing 18 inches to 24 inches in front of the cane tip. Studies have shown that this distance is ample enough to give the user time to evade tree branches, signs, and awnings which he normally has no way of detecting.

Ten laser canes have been delivered to the Veterans Administration, and have been tested by blind veterans. The VA has ordered an additional 35 canes for further testing. Presently, the cost of each cane is about $3,000, but the manufacturer hopes that once the canes go into full-scale production, the price can be reduced to about $1,000.

Laser canes are made by Bionic Instruments, Inc., of Bala Cynwyd, Pennsylvania.

71. STUTTERING GOES WITH TICKTOCK

IN THE PAST, only three out of every 10 persons who stuttered were able to be cured. Today, roughly four out of five stutterers can be cured with behavioral therapy treatment through *metronome-conditioned speech retraining*. The new procedure was developed by Dr. John Paul Brady at the University of Pennsylvania.

The new method is different from most psychiatric therapy in that it treats the stuttering directly, instead of trying to uncover psychological reasons for stuttering.

Metronome-conditioned speech retraining is accomplished in three phases. In phase one, the patient is taught to speak rhythmically with a standard metronome. During phase two, a miniaturized, electronic hearing aid size metronome is worn in public and substituted for the standard metronome. In the last phase, the patient is weaned from the mechanical devices.

The new therapy is routinely used by Dr. Perry A. Berman, a Philadelphia psychiatrist, many of whose patients have been failures in treatment by psychoanalysis, hypnosis, and other methods of treatment.

Treatment begins with Dr. Berman finding out how much the patient stutters and which situations are most difficult for him. (Many stutterers don't stutter when they're alone and are talking to themselves, or when they speak to a pet or a close friend, but they do stutter when they are suddenly

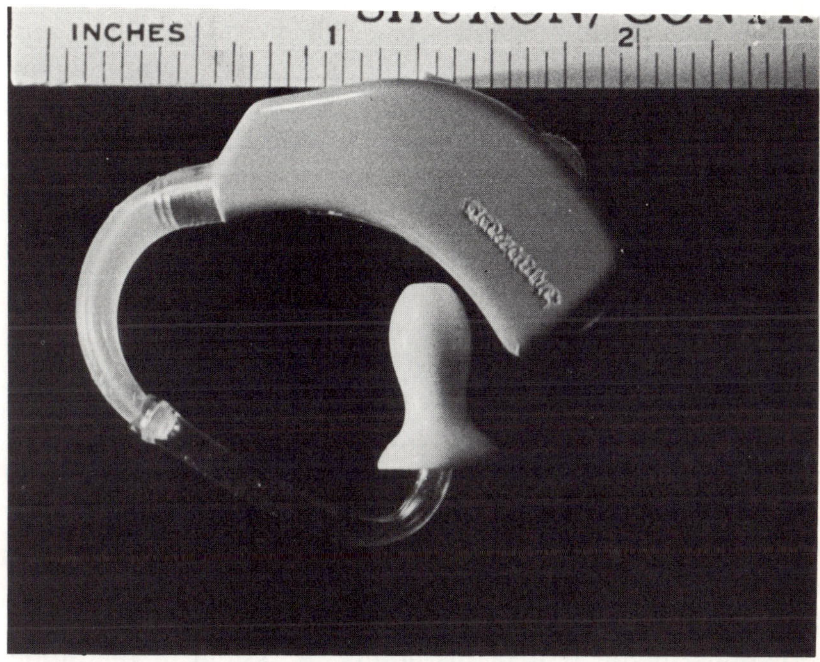

An electronic metronome

placed in a situation in which they *must* speak—a phone rings and they have to answer it, when they have to order food in a restaurant, or when they have to make a report to a boss.) A set of 8 or 10 stutter situations which are most difficult for the patient is set up by Dr. Berman.

The rhythmic speech training starts with the use of a common metronome. The ticktock regulates the number of syllables the patient utters in a minute. During the first hour of treatment, the metronome is slowed to a range of 40 to 80 beats a minute, depending on the patient's ability to speak his syllables fluently. The beat is gradually increased as the therapy progresses. At the end of the first week the rate may reach 100 to 120 a minute, during the second week about 130, and so on, up to 140-160. The therapy consists of weekly office visits and daily home practice.

The metronome-regulated speech is monotonous and machine-like, but the stuttering becomes less severe, and during the month or so of phase one, Dr. Berman teaches the patient to shape his speech to the beat of the metronome by uttering several syllables—or complete words—to one beat. Phase one ends with relatively normal sounding, but rhythmic speech.

During phase two—which may take four to five months—the patient wears the earpiece metronome, which looks like a hearing aid. It can even be fitted into eyeglasses.

The patient starts his public training with the easiest of the stutter situations set out for him by Dr. Berman. This may simply be speaking with his wife. When he can handle that, he moves on to the next situation on the list, and so through the complete list of situations that may have induced his stutter. He continues to come in for office visits during which time Dr. Berman guides him as he acts out the most difficult situations to the best of his ability. A system of relaxation therapy and systematic desensitization is then used.

In phase three, he starts to go through the stutter situations without the electronic pacer, again starting with the easiest situation. (In this stage, he is still using the earpiece for the more difficult situations.) After about six months and some 15 office sessions, the average patient no longer needs the metronome to help him speak normally under most conditions. Some stutterers, however, continue to use the earpiece in very difficult situations.

Although many psychological explanations exist to explain the reasons for stuttering, Dr. Berman does not find it useful to track them down in order to treat patients effectively. Often, the original cause has totally disappeared.

72. TREATMENT FOR THE DIABETIC'S FEET

ALTHOUGH MOST DIABETICS, especially those with adult diabetes (a form of diabetes which does not usually occur before the age of 40), can live normal, healthy lives, others, despite proper treatment, develop serious complications. Sometimes, severe premature arteriosclerosis attacks the coronary arteries, leading to a heart attack. The blood vessels of the legs may also be affected, producing difficulty in walking and eventually leading to painful ulcers and infections of the feet. In such cases, gangrene sometimes develops and a foot may have to be amputated.

If the "diabetic foot" results as a combination of impaired blood supply, infection and a disease of the nerves, the chances of saving the foot are not good.

Treatment for diabetics' feet has been studied extensively by Dr. Fred W. Whitehouse, Chief of the Division of Metabolic Diseases at the Henry Ford Hospital in Detroit. Foot trouble is a significant problem in diabetic patients, reports Dr. Whitehouse, pointing out that of the 541 consecutive diabetic patients seen by him over a ten-month period, 89 (16%) had some kind of a foot problem, 52 of them active problems demanding treatment. Of those, 17 had the

Additional material touching on this subject can be found in chapters 3, 19, 62 and 63.

diabetic foot caused by a combination of problems mentioned above and 10 of them lost their limbs.

Of the various problems, the most serious is the blocking of the blood vessels. But it is not easy for the doctor to determine whether the veins or the artery are blocked. If this can be determined, angioplasty (surgical repair of blood vessels) might be possible and the circulation of the blood restored. To determine where the vessels are blocked, the doctor does an aortogram. A colored fluid is injected into the aorta and then the leg is X-rayed. The colored fluid is visible on x-rays and shows where the blood vessels are blocked.

However, many doctors consider any form of corrective surgery unnecessarily risky in a diabetic and hesitate to do aortograms in these patients. Dr. Whitehouse is of a different opinion. In a selected group of diabetic patients at the Henry Ford Hospital, more than 100 have had aortography in a period of less than three years and it appears that about half of them had potentially operable conditions. Not all of these operable cases underwent angioplasty, but in those that did, the procedure was successful in eradicating the major complaint in nearly three fourths of the cases. Dr. Whitehouse believes that perhaps a third of these patients would have lost a foot if angioplasty had not been carried out.

73. SEALING TEETH
TO PREVENT DECAY

A NEW TECHNIQUE to prevent tooth decay is now beginning to be employed by dentists throughout the country. It is called pit and fissure sealing, and it calls for the application of a protective coating to the surfaces of the teeth.

The technique was first developed by Dr. Michael G. Buonocore of the Eastman Dental Center in Rochester, New York. Dr. Buonocore developed an adhesive sealing compound, called Nuva-Seal, which he applied with a fine brush to the chewing surfaces of the back teeth. After the sealant was spread on the surface of the teeth, it was then hardened to a glass-like solid with a hand-held ultraviolet lamp. This sealed the pits and fissures against any decay.

Pits and fissures are tiny indentations and grooves on the chewing surfaces of back teeth. They are actually defects in the tooth enamel which are common to normal teeth. (Front teeth usually have smooth enamel surfaces.) These pits and fissures are the spots where much of the dental decay occurs, particularly in children and adolescents. The enamel at these points is often thin and difficult to clean thoroughly. The bristles of a toothbrush cannot reach the tiny depressions. The sealant forms a coating on the grinding surfaces of the teeth, closing up the pits and fissures.

Dr. Buonocore found that two years after an application the sealant was 99% effective for reducing caries (decay) in adult

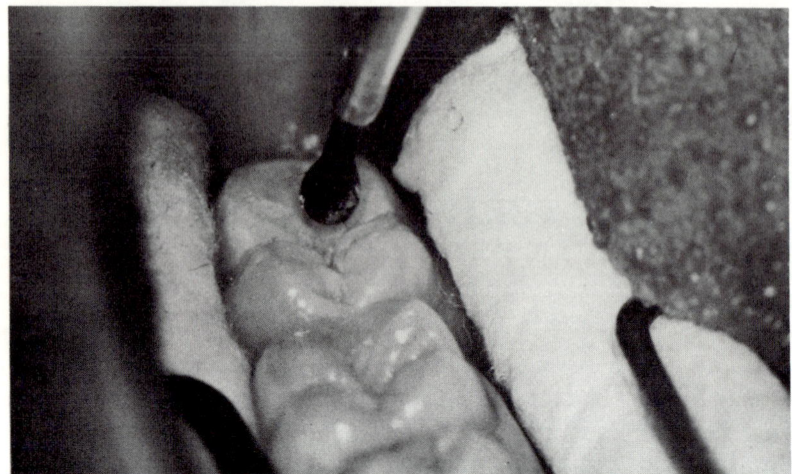

A drop of Nuva-Seal adhesive sealant being applied to a tooth surface.

teeth, and 87% effective for deciduous (baby) teeth. A group of patients who were used to compare the results of the sealed teeth with únprotected teeth, developed caries in 60% of unprotected adult teeth and in 38% of baby teeth. As some of the sealant had worn off during the two years, a re-application would have been needed to continue the protection.

Various sealants have been developed and are now being use by dentists, but only one, the Nuva-Seal, has been recognized (as of March, 1973) as an accepted restorative by the American Dental Association. The A.D.A. cautions that the new technique is one of *preventive* dentistry, and is *not* intended to replace regular oral hygiene. It is something to be used *in addition* to it.

The sealing procedure is painless and simple. The teeth are cleaned and dried. The sealant is then applied to each tooth and dried with the ultraviolet light. It only takes about three minutes for each tooth to be protected.

With the various dentists doing the new procedure, the best way to find out who is doing it in your local area is by asking your local dental society.

74. BRAIN FREEZE
FOR STROKE VICTIMS

EVERY YEAR nearly half a million Americans fall victim to strokes, and a large number of them are left with paralysis on one side of the body. This form of paralysis is called *spastic hemiplegia:* the arm and the leg on one side of the body become twisted, rigid and useless. Sometimes, this is accompanied by uncontrollable movements of the useless limbs and by loss of speech. Spastic hemiplegia can be excruciatingly painful.

Spastic hemiplegia also affects some victims of cerebral palsy as well as others who are stricken with certain types of brain tumors.

In the past, very little could be done to relieve this condition, but now, Dr. Irving S. Cooper, director of neurologic surgery at the St. Barnabas Hospital in New York City, developed a new surgical technique for treating spastic hemiplegia that often restores full use of the paralyzed limbs.

The new method is called *cryopulvinectomy* and it involves partial destruction of a brain structure called the *pulvinar*. The destruction is performed by freezing.

The pulvinar is a marble-sized region in the rear of the *thalamus,* a large, grey mass located in mid-brain, directly over the brain-end of the spinal cord. The functions of the pulvinar are not known, but it apparently acts as the central brain switchboard that has much to do with regulating movement.

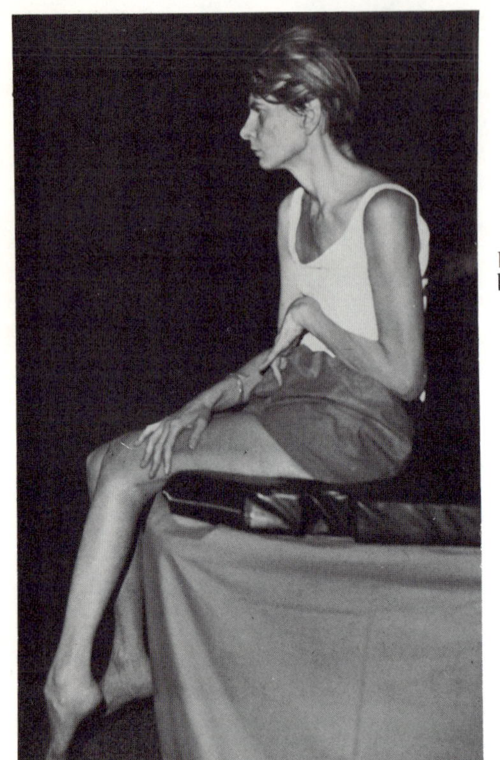

Distorted limbs (left) are straightened
by a cryopulvinectomy (below).

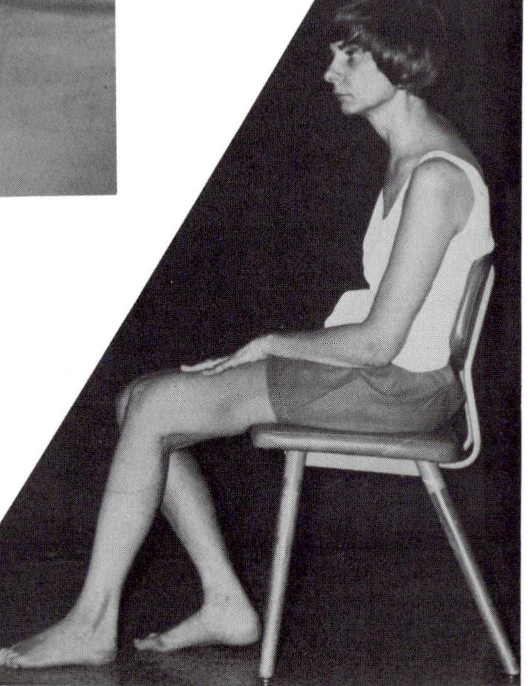

Dr. Cooper has been performing pioneering surgery in the thalamus region for 20 years, relieving the tremors of Parkinson's disease and treating various movement disorders. It was this work that led him to discover that the destruction of a part of the pulvinar will bring a dramatic relief in many cases of spastic hemiplegia.

In the past two years, Dr. Cooper has performed cryopulvinectomies on some 80 patients. Using a slender cryoprobe—a tube filled with liquid nitrogen—he probes the brain until the X-ray monitor shows that he has reached the pulvinar. Then, a press of a button on the cryoprobe reduces the temperature at its tip to minus 120 degrees centigrade. Several minutes are required to freeze and destroy carefully selected parts of the pulvinar. During the operation —which is painless—the patient is alert and wide awake.

If the operation is successful, the patient's twisted and rigid limbs—which sometimes have been rigid for years—instantly uncurl and relax. Further destruction of the pulvinar may be needed, and two or three more operating sessions may be required, but this additional surgery can often completely relieve the paralysis and restore the long-lost functions to the limbs.

To date, Dr. Cooper reports that he has brought significant relief of paralysis and restored motor functions to about 60 percent of the patients he has operated on. The effects of the operation on those who were previously totally incapacitated are of extreme importance. "The benefit to the patient and his family is inestimable," says Dr. Cooper, "if I can get voluntary muscle control in even one limb."

In the future, Dr. Cooper estimates the success rate should be much higher. He bases his optimism on the probability of the development of more exact screening methods to determine which patients can benefit from cryopulvinectomy.

75. MEASURING EYE PULSE
    TO DETERMINE ARTERY HEALTH

A NEW YORK DOCTOR has devised a way of measuring the pulse of the eye in order to check the state of health of the arteries which supply blood to the head and brain.

The problem involved here was the measurement of the flow of blood—always a difficult procedure despite the many new techniques now available to doctors.

Accurate measurement of the flow of blood always involves painful procedures and cannot be carried out on a person in poor general condition, the aged, or those suffering from various heart diseases. The new technique, invented by Dr. Miles A. Galin, of the New York Medical College in Manhattan, is safe and painless—and ingenious.

The eye, being an organ that is heavily supplied with arteries and veins, pulsates in response to the pressures of blood which surge through it—as does every other organ of the body. To measure its pulse, Dr. Galin devised a tiny plastic suction cup which he applies to the side of the eye, after it has been anesthesized. The water-filled cup is connected to a transducer which senses the tiny changes in pressure on the eye and converts them into electrical signals. These signals are then fed to a computer for storage and analysis. When the information is needed, the computer prints out a graph.

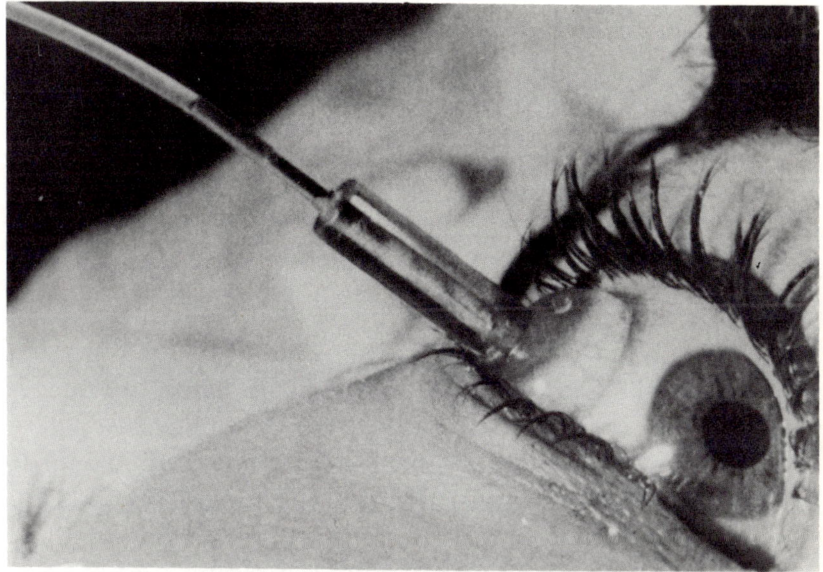

A suction cup being used to monitor ocular pulse.

After Dr. Galin perfected the system in the laboratory, he tried it on 22 patients suspected of having plugged carotid arteries (those which run up the neck on each side of the throat to feed blood to the brain and head).

By analyzing the graphs produced by the computer for each eye, he could determine if one carotid artery or both was open or was obstructing the flow of blood. Since some of the cases of plugged carotid arteries cannot be determined safely and easily with present-day techniques, the new technique of the eye pulse measurements promises to be an important medical tool which will make these difficult determinations now possible in persons whose state of health previously barred them from such examinations.

76. A PACIFIER FOR STOMACH PAINS

THE CONDITION called by doctors "bile reflux gastritis" is a very distressing situation. The afflicted is subject to a persistent, unrelenting, severe stomach pain which radiates up to the lower chest. After eating, the pain becomes worse and antacids are of no help. Appetite is down, and many of those stricken with this condition lose a lot of weight. Most of them frequently vomit a bitter fluid, and many suffer from distressing diarrhea. Sometimes, the symptoms become so severe as to be disabling.

The malady afflicts men and women alike, and can occur at almost any age in an adult. The reasons for the condition vary, and it may be chronic or acute, but the chronic type is quite common. Various diseases of the stomach may be associated with this condition, a common one being an ulcer.

Stomach surgery often predisposes one to this problem. The main cause of the condition is probably bile splashing up into the stomach. This is the opinion of Dr. Harold H. Scudamore, of the Monroe Clinic, in Monroe, Wisconsin. Dr. Scudamore also believes that emotional stress is a factor in a number of cases.

Dr. Scudamore has been treating patients with bile reflux gastritis by giving them a drug called *cholestyramine*. It is dissolved in orange juice, and taken one hour after each meal and at bedtime. Dr. Scudamore has treated 42 patients with bile reflux gastritis, all chronic sufferers from this condition. His patients have ranged in age from 25 to 75; half of them men and half women.

Of these 42 patients, nine had persistent diarrhea; 19 had previous stomach surgery; eight had ulcers; three also had cancer, and most of them were persistently vomiting. Most of them have had these symptoms for several years. Some of them were treated by surgery, but 20 received cholestyramine. Of these 20, 10 responded favorably, and four showed fair improvement.

Patients usually improved within one to two weeks. Some of them have now been on the drug a year and have not suffered any side effects.

Dr. Scudamore believes that cholestyramine is the most beneficial treatment in mild cases of bile reflux gastritis, and that it is particularly beneficial in cases involving diarrhea. As a side benefit, cholestyramine also helps to heal gastric ulcers.

77. THE CLOSEST THING
TO A REAL HAND

MOST AMPUTEES have not even heard of a *myoelectric hand*, but this new artificial hand is destined to replace the artificial hands now in use.

Compared to an ordinary artificial hand, the myoelectric hand is like comparing a modern automobile to a horse-and-buggy. It is really a dream come true. An artificial hand which works exactly like a real hand! It can grasp, lift, squeeze—and if two are worn, each works independently of the other. The user can hold a piece of bread in one hand and butter it with the other. It *looks* just like a real hand, too.

The myoelectric hand—properly called a *myoelectrically controlled prosthesis*—was developed in Italy by Mr. Hannes Schmidl, an Austrian-born prosthetist, who first started to work on the idea in 1963, after having been invited to work in Italy by the Italian National Insurance Institute for Industrial Accidents (INAIL). By the spring of 1964, Schmidl and his team manufactured the world's first two myoelectric hands. The patents on the hand are held by the Italian government, thus insuring that no personal profit will accrue to anyone from Schmidl's invention—which is as he wanted it.

The myoelectric hand works by electricity in the human body. Whenever a person flexes his muscle, the movement produces an electric discharge in the body. This signal is very

Additional material touching on this subject can be found in chapter 63.

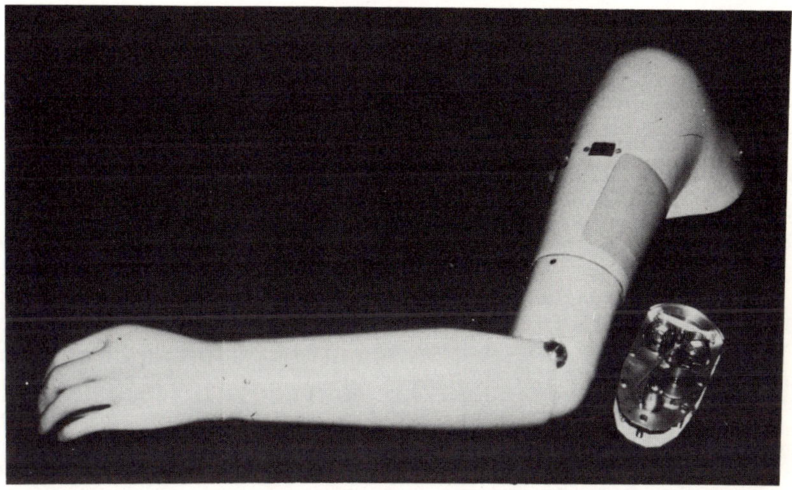

A myoelectric arm with an exposed elbow unit.

weak. A moving muscle produces only one-thousandth of a volt of electricity, which is watered down to one-millionth of a volt by the time it reaches the surface of the skin. This signal is picked up by metal skin contacts of the prosthesis and is amplified some 50 thousand times to turn on the artificial hand's small, battery-powered motor.

In addition to the motor, the hand is equipped with a gear box which, like the automatic transmission in a car, provides the variations in "speeds" needed to move the fingers and the wrist at the proper pace. The control is so effective that the hand is able to lift a chair, or cut a steak, or handle a pair of tweezers.

In addition to the artificial hand, Schmidl also developed a myoelectric arm suitable to be worn by above-elbow amputees. The artificial arm permits hand opening and closing, wrist rotation and elbow flexion (bending) and extension—all at the same time, each synchronized with the others, just like in a real arm. An experienced wearer of the new artificial arm can grasp with his hand, and at the same time, turn his wrist and bend his elbow.

The artificial hand works by moving the muscles in the arm —as if a real hand were attached to the end of it. But, with the artificial arm, there are no muscles to move and the armless patient must think or pretend that he is moving muscles which he no longer has in order to produce the correct electric signal.

The artificial arm has several motors inside, duplicating eight of the sixteen basic movements of the human arm from the shoulder to the fingers. The skin contacts receive signals from four major muscles in the shoulder, and, using signals produced by various levels of muscle effort, eight signals are obtained from only four muscles.

The INAIL myoelectric hand and arm are now available in the United States. The Institute of Rehabilitation Medicine in New York City has been licensed by INAIL to adapt the system to their patients. The Institute is now fully equipped as a *myoelectric prosthetic fitting center*. The cost of the myoelectric hand ranges from $2,000.00 for a hand to $4,000.00 for a full arm.

78. IMPROVING SPEECH
WITH TEFLON VOCAL CORDS

TRY AS THEY MAY, many persons can't talk above a whisper. Their voice problems have many origins. Some have had vocal cords or nerves damaged in car accidents. Others acquire a problem after a *thoractomy* (any operation involving an incision in the wall of the chest), or it may come as the result of a thyroid operation.

The problem that develops is that one vocal cord is not in the midline: air escapes, and speech is often almost impossible. In addition, there is very real danger of aspiration (drawing out, by suction, fluid from other body cavities, such as, for example, the chest).

These sufferers from assorted vocal problems can now be helped with injections of Teflon into the vocal cord. It's the same Teflon which makes things super smooth and is used to coat kitchen frying pans and bridge sections.

The idea is not new. Sixty years ago, a German surgeon successfully treated patients by injecting hard paraffin (which also makes things smooth) into paralyzed vocal cords. However, paraffin injections were dropped when it was discovered that they produced dangerous side effects.

The Teflon injections were recently reported on by Dr. Herbert Dedo, Associate Professor of Otolaryngology at the

---

Additional material touching on this subject can be found in chapters 5 and 41.

University of California in San Francisco, who administered them to 135 patients. According to Dr. Dedo, the results were striking, with many patients starting to talk and cry right in the operating room.

Of the 135 patients, 81% recovered their normal voice, and 97% improved. Aspiration was decreased or completely eliminated in the majority of patients. Only four of the 135 patients did not improve at all, and all of them had voice problems relating to severe surgery and accidents.

In the actual procedure, Dr. Dedo injects the Teflon into the vocal cord and, as he does it, he asks the patients to speak. The voice changes from a breathy, weak, hoarse speech to a clear, firm voice in a majority of cases.

According to Dr. Dedo, the Teflon injections are a good answer to what has been a very difficult problem. "What we are really doing," says Dr. Dedo, "is tuning the vocal cords with Teflon."

79. MIGRAINE CONTROL THROUGH BIOFEEDBACK

BIOFEEDBACK TRAINING is a process of learning to become aware of involuntary (automatic) changes within a person's body and of learning how to control them.

The person undergoing biofeedback training is wired to a machine and is told by its beeps, or by a wavering needle, just what his brain or heart is up to. He then tries, by a process of trial and error, to control his heartbeat, brainwaves, blood pressure, etc. The machine tells him if he is succeeding.

Once a person trains himself to control a specific action of his body, such as, for example, regulating the heartbeat or lowering the blood pressure, he can then learn to control these actions anytime he wishes without the aid of the machine.

Doctors in many research centers throughout the country are working with biofeedback to learn what ailments can be controlled through this training. Dr. Elmer Green, at the Menninger Foundation, in Topeka, Kansas, has taught his patients to control their migraines—those blinding, often incapacitating superheadaches, which come and go, and from which there is often no relief.

Control of body temperature is the key in the biofeedback migraine control. Patients who can learn from the machine to raise the temperature of their fingers higher than that of their

---

Additional material touching on this subject can be found in chapters 48, 57, 67, 79, 85 and 91.

head temperature, can prevent migraine attacks.

In training sessions, the patients sit facing a small, transistor-radio-sized machine with temperature sensors taped to their foreheads and to one forefinger. They are instructed to "think" their hands are warm. On the first few tries, usually nothing happens, but after some practice most of them learn to raise the temperature in their fingers by thinking them warm.

Actually, what they are doing is increasing blood circulation in their hands. Why this increase of blood circulation in the hand stops migraine is not a complete mystery, though exactly how it works is unknown. The theory is that migraine is caused by dilation of blood vessels in the head, which results in pressure on nerves and causes headaches. Directing the flow of blood towards the hands, might be diverting it from the blood vessels in the head and thus prevent their dilation—and, consequently, prevent migraine headaches.

Biofeedback is also being used to control high blood pressure and a variety of common ailments, such as tension headaches, asthma attacks, and irregular heartbeat, and insomnia. It is still in the research stage and it training should be done only under direct supervision of a physician.

There are many portable biofeedback devices on the market today, so-called "alpha control" machines, and they have been advertised and suggested as means of controlling all kinds of ailments, including alcoholism and drug addiction. The use of these machines without a doctor's supervision cannot be recommended.

80. BRINGING RELIEF
TO THE GREAT TOE

THE GREAT TOE is subject to many painful and disabling conditions, the most common of them being caused by *rheumatoid arthritis* or *osteoarthritis*. These two types of arthritis erode the joints of the toes causing them to twist painfully over each other. Normal walking becomes impossible.

Two other fairly common deformities of the big toe—*hallux valgus* and *hallux rigidus*—can be very painful and disabling. The first is a condition in which the big toe deviates towards the other side of the foot; the second, known as "stiff toe," is caused by a stiffness in the joint where the big toe joins the foot.

These three conditions can now be corrected by implanting an artificial joint in the great toe. The artificial joint is made of silicone rubber, and was invented by Dr. Alfred B. Swanson of Blodgett Memorial Hospital, Grand Rapids, Michigan. Dr. Swanson has developed a series of silicone rubber implants for various joints in the body, and has pioneered the operations in which they are implanted. His various artificial joints, and his operating techniques, are used throughout the world. The most commonly used, are for the finger joints. The artificial joint for the big toe is his latest development.

Additional material touching on this subject can be found in chapters 3, 62, 63 and 72.

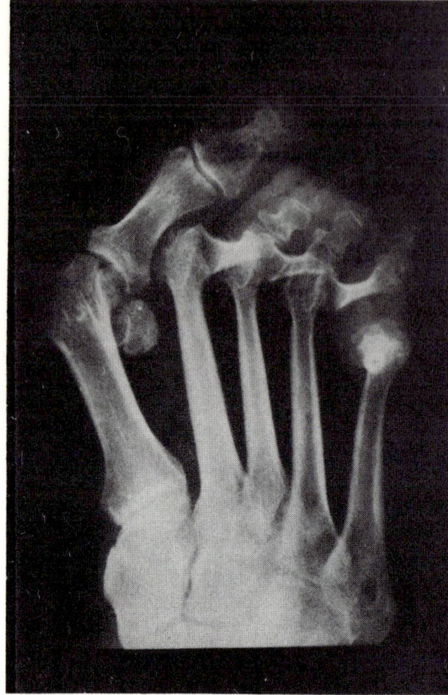

An X-ray of the toes of a 59 year-old woman with rhematoid arthritis before the implant of an artificial joint.

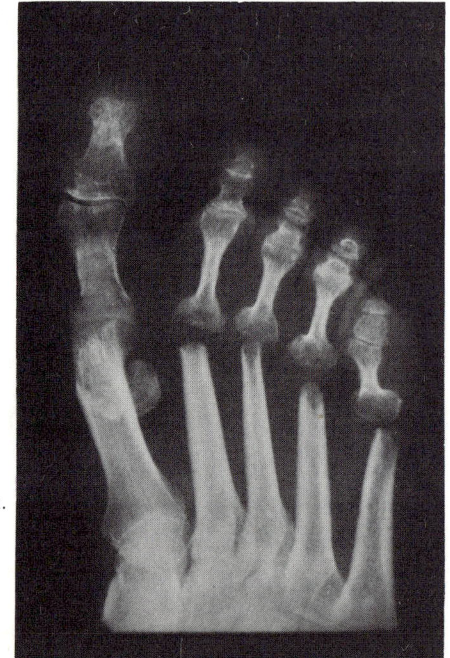

The same toes two years after implantation.

The artificial joints are made by the Dow Corning Corporation, Midland, Michigan, and the joints for the big toe are tested on an ingenious machine which simulates the action of the joint in order to test the stress resistance of the implant. The implant was tested through a simulation of 250,000,000 stress movements—equivalent to walking ten times around the globe.

In the actual procedure, the joints of the big toe are exposed through an incision, and the ends of the second joint are trimmed to obtain a smooth and rounded surface. If the bones are too long, or deformed, they are shortened and reshaped.

The artificial joint, which looks like a button with a stem (see photos), is implanted by inserting the stem into the second bone of the big toe (the bone has a canal which is shaped to receive the stem with a special drill). The reason that the implant is introduced at the base of the second phalanx is that this is the part of the big toe which bears only minimal weight, and this makes the reconstructed joint free of heavy stress.

A few days after the operation, a special splint is applied to the great toe in order to keep it in alignment while allowing the toes to exercise and strengthen the muscles. The splint is worn continuously for 3-4 weeks and then used as a night splint for approximately 3-6 weeks. The patient may walk on his heel in a week.

During the past four years, Dr. Swanson has implanted the artificial joint in 117 great toes with excellent results. His patients range in age from 17 to 79, and 31 of them had the artificial joint implanted in the great toes of both feet. The patients have all remarked about the minimum amount of pain during the postoperative period, and all have been pleased with the results.

81. PLASTIC IMPLANT
CORRECTS CHEST DEPRESSION

PECTUS EXCAVATUS, a birth defect involving an ugly depression in the breast bone, can now be corrected by inserting artificial material under the skin to fill the depression.

Though the defect in itself is not dangerous to one's health and seldom causes complications requiring surgery, it is an unpleasant condition which causes those afflicted a great deal of embarrassment. They are often reluctant to swim or engage in sports without a shirt on.

The cause of this birth defect is unknown. The number of afflicted persons is about one out of every 2,500 births, the exact figures being difficult to come by, since only the most severe cases are operated on; the rest going by unnoticed.

Operations to correct this condition in the past have involved cutting the ribs and breast bone, entering the heart and lung cavities, and repositioning the bone and cartilage of the front wall of the chest. These operations were long and dangerous. Serious complications and death resulted in a number of cases. The postoperative period was long and painful, and the results were often poor. In many cases, the scarring and irregularities brought little, if any, improvement in the person's appearance. As often as not, the operations failed to correct the defect, and the depression would re-appear.

Additional material touching on this subject can be found in chapter 26.

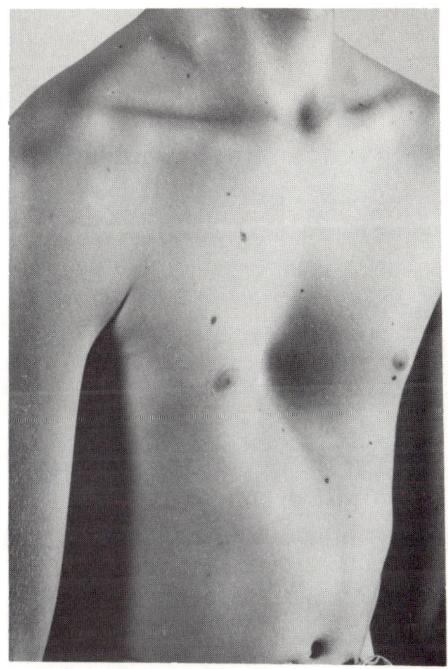

A view of a depressed breast bone before the corrective operation.

The same patient after the implant.

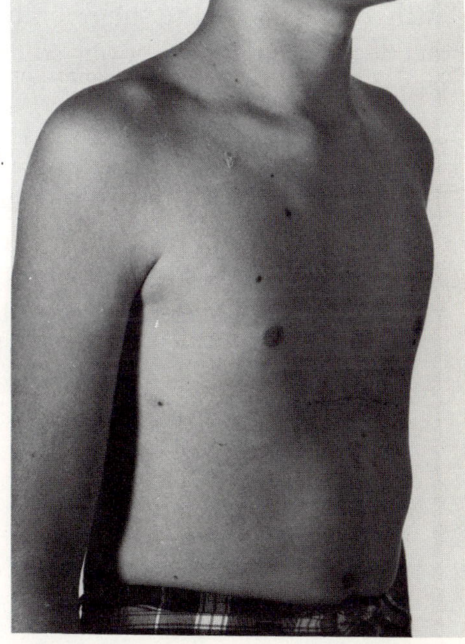

The new implant technique was devised by Colonel David G. Bowers, Jr., of the Wilford Hall U.S. Air Force Medical Center, Lackland Air Force Base, Texas. It is simple, safe, and sometimes can even be done under local anesthesia. It leaves a much smaller and less visible scar than that of any other procedure.

The plastic implant is custom-made to fit the depression in the patient's chest a few days before the actual operation. It is made by moulding the material right on the chest so that it fits the depression exactly.

To insert the implant, the surgeon makes a slit in the skin of the chest. Because both the implant and the skin are flexible, the incision is short. The implant's edges are folded under, slipped in under the skin, opened up, and positioned in the depression. The incision is then closed. When healing is complete, only a short scar remains.

The operation takes less than one hour. Since there is very little bleeding during the operation, a blood transfusion is not needed. None of the serious complications common to the old procedures come into play.

Colonel Bowers has already used his procedure on nine patients ranging in age from 13 to 42 years. So far, all nine have been very pleased with the results. None of them has complained of any restrictions in movement or in any of their normal activities. The weight of the implant has not presented a problem to any of the patients.

The 13-year-old boy has had the implant now three years.

82. NEW TREATMENT FOR WILSON'S DISEASE

WILSON'S DISEASE is an inherited, progressive disease caused by excessive accumulation of copper in the body, particularly in the brain, liver, cornea and kidneys. The disease is slow in progress, but it is deadly. It is also very difficult to diagnose correctly because its first symptoms are almost exactly the same as those of chronic hepatitis.

The human body needs various minerals to perform its many functions. They are eaten along with food and though many are needed in a very tiny amount—some in millionths of an ounce—all are essential in the proper amounts. Minerals needed include copper, cobalt, zinc, manganese and molybendum—called the essential trace minerals. An average man possesses a total of about 1/28th of an ounce of these five minerals. However, the minerals must be processed by the body in a manner that allows only the needed amounts to be retained in the system. Sometimes, the body fails to do this properly and accumulates too much of a given mineral. One such mineral which sometimes accumulates in excess quantities is copper.

The excessive accumulations of copper in the body are caused by faulty copper metabolism. This excess accumulation of copper begins at birth, during which time copper accumulates in the bile. There may be no symptoms of any illness at this stage, which shifts or blends into the next stage in which liver failure is common—and fatal. During this stage, some of the patients develop a tell-tale symptom of the disease called the Kayser-Fleischer rings—greenish-yellow rings in the eyes, caused by accumulation of copper in the corneas.

If the patient survives the second stage, he may again revert to stage one—apparently free of illness. However, he continues to accumulate copper, but now, instead of accumulating it in the bile, he accumulates it in the brain. After a period of time, the victim enters a stage of neurologic disease, accompanied by clearly visible Kayser-Fleischer rings, tremors, spasticity, trouble in speaking and swallowing, and cirrhosis of the liver. Death follows shortly.

The conventional treatment for this condition has been the use of drugs which prevent the build-up of copper in the body and which increase its excretion in bile. One of these drugs, potassium sulfide, has been in use since 1954; the other, penicillamine, was first introduced in 1956.

Now, Dr. G. E. Cartwright, of the University of Utah College of Medicine, at Salt Lake City, has published the first results of long-term treatments with penicillamine of a group of Wilson's Disease patients. These patients have been on the drug from 9 to 13 years and observations made by Dr. Cartwright over the period of these years convincingly show that this type of treatment is precisely what is needed by the afflicted. The long period of observation has shown that the drug must be administered at all times, because as soon as it is withheld, the copper begins to accumulate again. On the other hand, while under treatment, and continuously taking penicillamine, a person with Wilson's Disease can lead a normal life.

The five patients who were the subject of this long study are all well and leading normal lives. Two work as clerks, one as a house painter, one as a housewife, and one as a college student. When they first started on the drug, three of the patients were severely incapacitated by neurologic disease. All three suffered from tremors and had difficulty in speaking. The fourth patient was psychotic, violent and abusive. The fifth patient was completely incapacitated, bedridden, mentally dull, and had to be fed through a stomach tube.

The recoveries were not instant. Tremors started to lessen in 18 to 24 months, and disappeared completely after 3 years, except for one patient whose tremors required six years on the drug to stop completely. Speech difficulties improved slowly over the period of years and one patient remained with a slight speech impairment even after 13 years. The violent patient recovered from psychosis within three months.

In a related study, researchers at the Albert Einstein College of Medicine in New York found that because Wilson's Disease so often may be taken for chronic hepatitis, many patients are incorrectly diagnosed and denied proper treatment for it. Instead they are treated for chronic hepatitis, which they don't have. These researchers strongly recommend that every young patient with chronic hepatitis be considered as a possible victim of Wilson's Disease and that he be examined for it to the point of either confirming that he has it or definitely eliminating that possibility.

83. "TALKING" EXERCISER FOR CHILDREN WITH CEREBRAL PALSY

A NEW THERAPEUTIC exerciser, which is both fun and beneficial for children suffering from cerebral palsy, is now being introduced.

Called Peter Pachyderm, the exerciser is designed to look like a stuffed toy. A soft, stain-resistant, plush elephant head with big floppy ears, short plastic tusks and two huge feet below it is attached to the front of the exerciser. The elephant is tan and brown, with white tusks and toes. Tusks can be removed and reattached.

A tape recorder, fitted into a compartment behind the elephant's head, is turned on by pushing a button in the tip of the trunk. Tapes which contain instructions, animal sounds or even a story, and which can be reached only by bending over, provide an incentive for the child to perform helpful exercises which may be painful. Suitable for children ages 3 to 14, the exerciser stretches and strengthens back, upper leg and hamstring muscles. Feet and knee supports hold the heel lift down and help to support the child's legs in a natural position.

The exerciser was designed by Chuck Flanigan, a graduate of San Jose State College's School of Industrial Design, and a winner in the Aluminum Company of America's Student Design competition.

Additional material touching on this subject can be found in chapter 100.

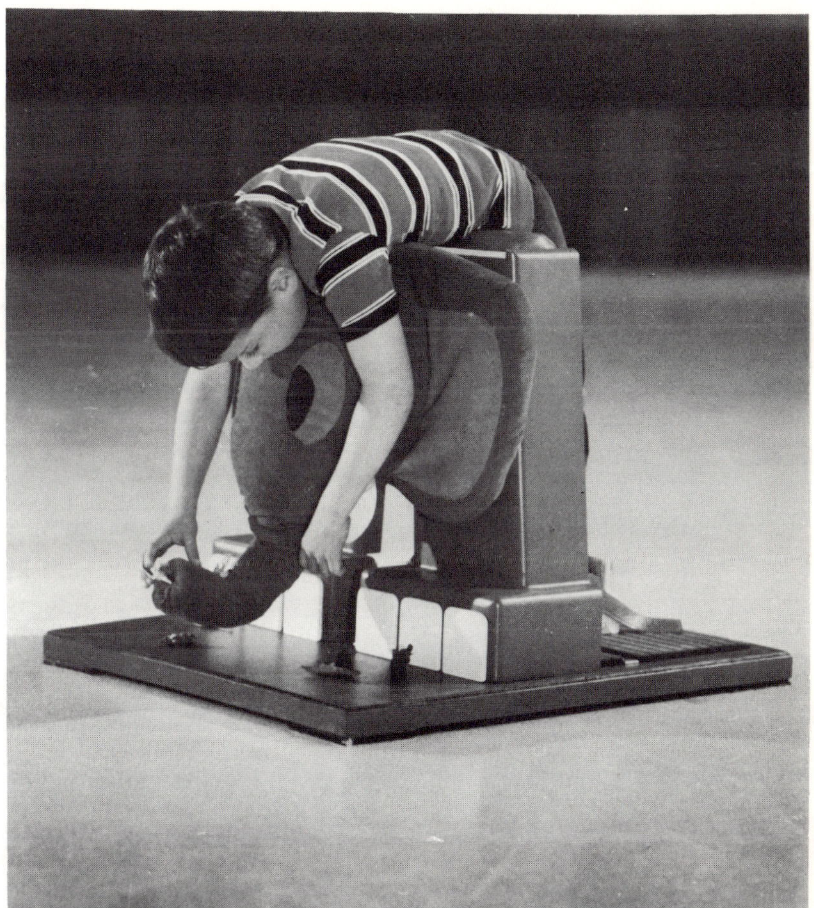

Peter Pachyderm in action. The photo shows how the child using the exerciser turns on the hidden tape recorder.

The exerciser was developed in conjunction with the Santa Clara Valley Medical Center and in consultations with therapists working with cerebral palsied children. It has important advantages over present methods. Until now, the therapist either had to support the child himself by wrapping his arms around the knees and ankles, thus putting a strain on himself, or he had to use awkward tilt tables which gave in-

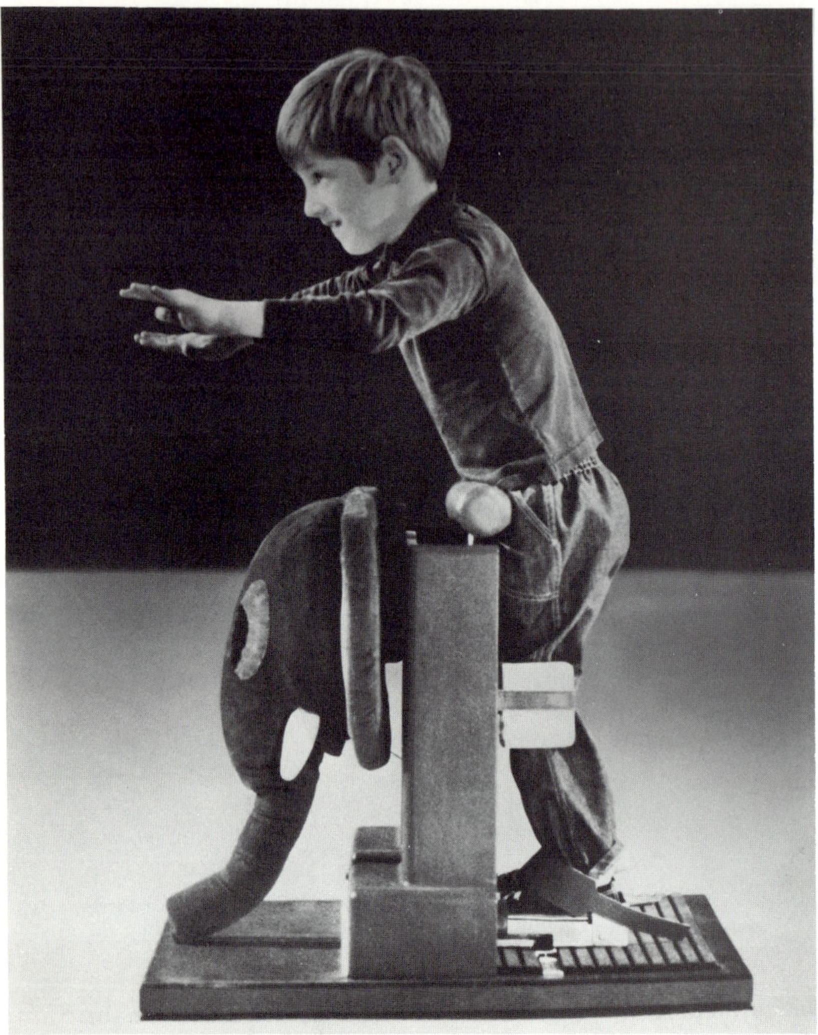

The palsy exerciser, showing how the child is securely held while in motion.

adequate leg support. The new exerciser supports the child securely and naturally.

The exerciser can be adapted to conform to body sizes of children ages 3 to 14. Feet, knee and abdominal supports are adjustable in one-inch increments. Legs may be positioned closely together or spread.apart, depending upon exercise requirements. Velcro fasteners on foot and knee supports provide a range of adjustments and make it easier to release the child. The waist band is secured by surcingle buckles.

The unit is mounted on a sturdy platform atop lockable casters which are spaced so that it is impossible to tip the exerciser by overbalancing it. Casters make the exerciser easily transportable, as is required by state fire codes.

The exerciser is priced at $350.00 plus shipping costs. It is made by the Overly Manufacturing Co., Greensburg, Pennsylvania.

84. NEW PACEMAKER INVENTED— WORKS VIA THE TELEPHONE

PATIENTS WHO DEPEND upon a cardiac pacemaker to assist their heart function will be encouraged to learn that a smaller, long-lived model has been approved for regular use, along with a companion transmitter for periodic checking of performance.

The new pacemaker-transmitter is the culmination of four years of research and evaluation by Dr. Albert Starr, of the University of Oregon Medical School, in collaboration with Edwards Laboratories in California.

Dr. Starr had two goals:

1. to try to extend the life of the pacemaker, which had been about two years, and

2. to develop a follow-up system.

The problem of following patients around the country with implanted pacemakers was increasing enormously, and these electronic instruments were crucial to the life of the patient.

These problems have been solved. The new pacemaker, activated on implant instead of at the time of manufacture, expends less energy with each stimulated pulse than did its predecessors, and is expected to last about 40 months.

The transmitter, which is given to the patient, picks up signals on two radio frequencies from the pacemaker. One in-

---

Additional material touching on this subject can be found in chapters 7, 24, 32, 46, 96, 98 and 99.

dicates the pacemaker is stimulating the heart, the other, that the heart is working by itself.

The doctor can now keep a closer check on the pacemaker's performance by having the patient phone him at one or two-month intervals, and through the telephone, send signals from the pacemaker to receiving equipment in the Medical school.

To check in by phone, the patient holds the transmitter next to his chest, over his implanted pacemaker. At the other end of this wire is a phone clip—which will fit any design of phone.

The Medical School has electronic receivers set up in its cardiac center where technicians take the calls. On the equipment in the cardiac center, sound signals from the transmitter are picked up and translated into visual signals: a yellow light tells the technician that the heart is operating on its own; a red one indicates that the pacemaker is working. The viewer also records the actual pulse rate.

A technician watches the viewer while he or she talks with the patient. Thus, if the pulse rate is slower than it should be, or if the patient reports dizziness or any other abnormal condition, the technician can take appropriate action. He may advise a visit to the doctor, send help if that seems indicated, or send a new transmitter if there appears to be no signal coming through.

The viewer can also be set up in any doctor's office. The telephone check-in can be made from anywhere in the world —cables are not necessary. A radio phone is equally suitable. The pacemaker currently costs around $900. So far, some 500 of them have already been implanted by cardiac surgeons.

85. AN ELECTRONIC PAIN KILLER

MANY AMERICANS suffer from pain so intense that they cannot work or even sleep. Drugs offer no relief. Now, an electronic device, called a *dorsal column stimulator*, is enabling some of them to lead normal lives.

A study conducted by a Long Beach, California neurosurgeon, Dr. Anselmo Pineda, on 45 patients suffering from chronic intractable (impossible to relieve) pain, revealed that 29 of them experienced excellent relief after he implanted the electronic device in their spinal columns. Another eight patients reported good pain relief.

The dorsal column stimulator works on the theory of blocking the pain impulses in the dorsal (back) section of the spinal column, before the pain can be transmitted to the brain where it is sensed.

The operation involves implanting an electrode—a hair-thin wire—into the spinal column, and connecting it to a radio receiving unit the size of a silver dollar. This device is placed under the skin of the patient's chest. The radio transmitting unit, outside the body, is the size of a cigarette package.

The technique is called *electroanalgesia*—pain relief from electrical stimulation. When a patient feels pain, he places the external, battery-powered transmitter and antenna directly

---

Additional material touching on this subject can be found in chapters 34 and 57.

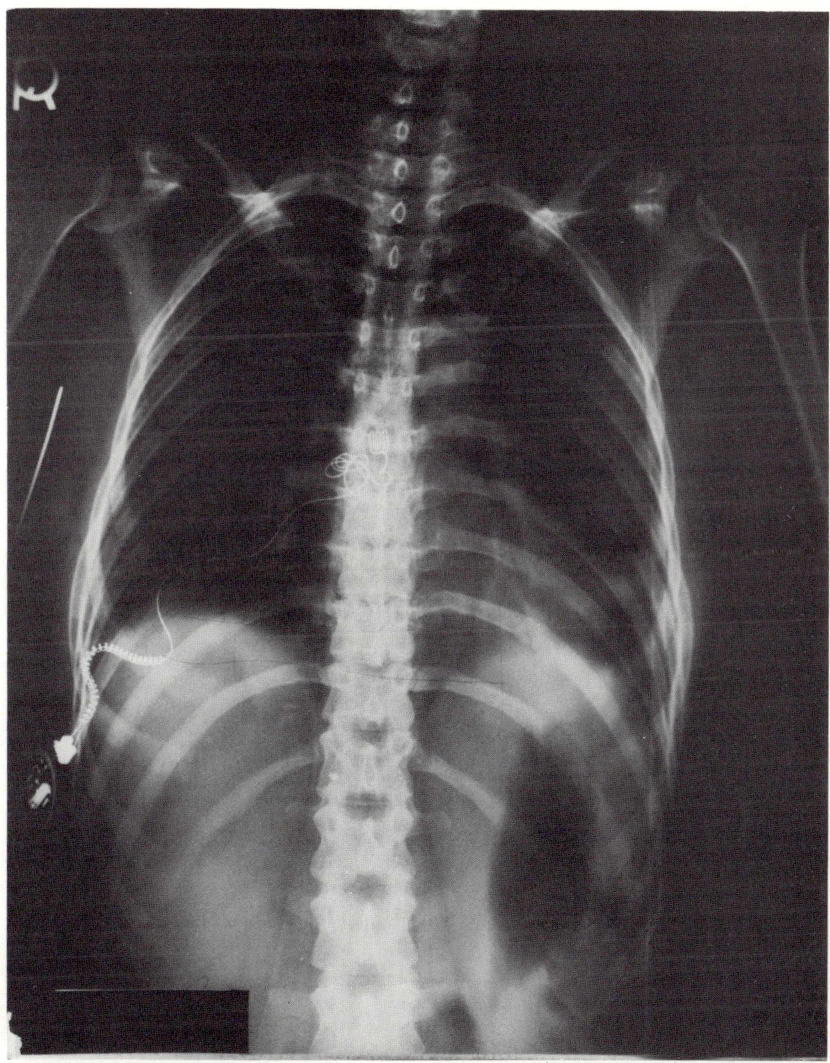

An X-ray showing an implanted dorsal column stimulator.

over the implanted receiver and turns on the radio current. The amount of time the device is used depends on how often the pain occurs and is controlled by the patient. Patients with constant pain leave the stimulator turned on even while sleeping.

The stimulator does not affect a person's sense of touch, and he experiences no difficulty in walking. There is no change in bladder or bowel control. Patients wearing the stimulator have continued their normal sexual activities. According to Dr. Pineda, the use of the stimulator does not affect a person's ability to think or his personality. (Patients relieved of long-standing pain, of course, may experience a dramatic change in their general outlook.)

Patients who have been helped by the implanatation of the dorsal column stimulator include those suffering from terminal cancer, those whose chronic pain was unrelieved by multiple spinal disc surgeries and sufferers of phantom limb distress and causalgia (a burning pain caued by an injury to a peripheral nerve).

Though the implantation of the device cannot be used for relief of all kinds of pain, it is, according to Dr. Pineda, "no longer considered experimental." However, he warns, "it should not be undertaken by those not completely familiar with, or trained in, the technique, which demands careful steps for successful results."

86. NEW SURGICAL TOOL
TO REMOVE HEMORRHOIDS

IF YOU ARE among the more than 63 million Americans who
suffer from hemorrhoids, chances are you seldom, if ever, discuss your ailment. What's more, many persons consider the
current surgical cure to be worse than suffering with the
hemorrhoids. Generally, they consent to surgery only as a last
resort.

A new method of surgically removing hemorrhoids has now
been developed that is taking away much of the pain (and, as
a consequence, the fear of pain) that has hitherto confronted
hemorrhoid operations.

Called *Kryostik,* and introduced by Sybron Corp. of
Rochester, N.Y., the new tool enables a physician to perform a
hemorrhoidectomy in his office. The procedure is usually
painless and quick. The patient can walk in and out of the
doctor's office the same day, and he will be able to return to
work the next morning. This, of course, means no hospital ex-
pense, and no lost pay because of absence from work.

Kryostik employs painless procedure and requires no spinal
or general anesthesia. The instrument provides its own
anesthetic through the extremely cold temperature
generated at the tip—the portion which touches tissue. All the
patient feels is a slight tingling sensation.

The *cryosurgical hemorrhoidectomy,* as the operation is
called medically, consists of touching the tip of the Kryostik to

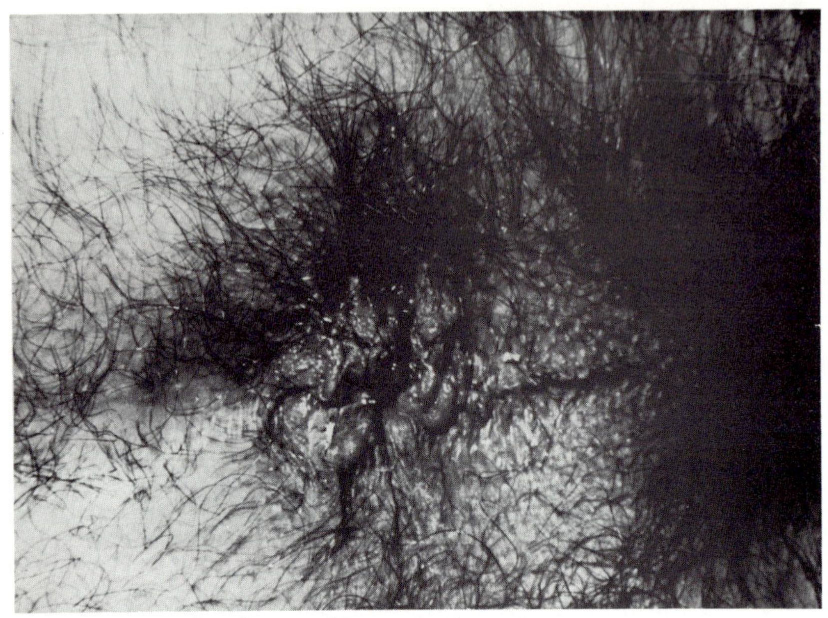

External and internal hemorrhoids producing severe pain.

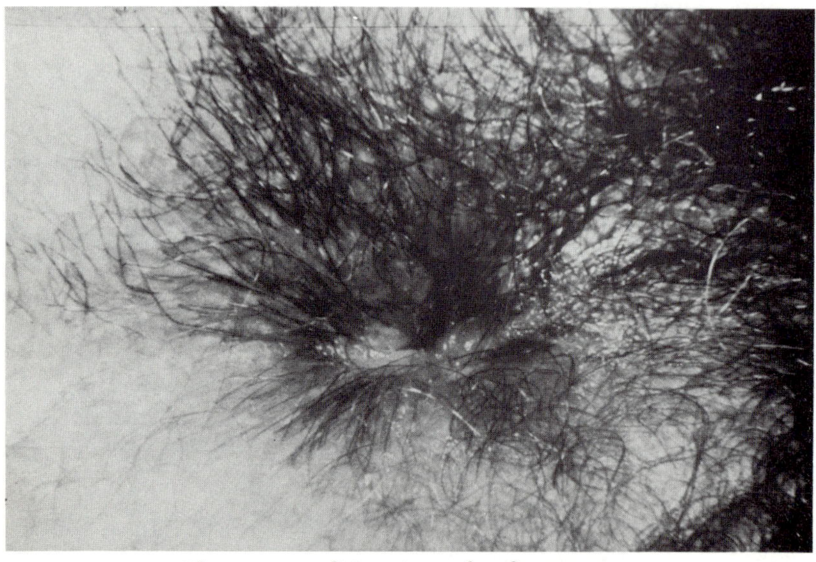

The same condition six weeks after surgery.

the hemorrhoid. The tissue freezes in a circular pattern at the point touched by the tip. Discoloration of the frozen tissue indicates to the physician the amount and extent of freezing. In cases of multiple hemorrhoids, each one must be touched individually to insure that all the swollen tissue is destroyed.

After the cryosurgery is complete, the patient wears a pad for about two weeks to absorb the frozen hemorrhoid tissue which sloughs off by itself.

Dr. Martin I. Lewis, the Hollywood, California physician who invented Kryostik, says that less than four per cent of his patients needed pain relieving medication following a Kryostik hemorrhoidectomy. "Even in those cases," he says, "the medication was necessary for only two or three days."

87. MECHANICAL ASSISTANCE TO THE FAILING HEART

AN INGENIOUS SURGICAL procedure, called intraaortic balloon pumping, is being increasingly used to fight cardiogenic shock, a condition which accounts for many in-hospital deaths from heart attack.

Out of some 600,00 victims of heart attack each year in the United States, 15 to 20 percent also suffer cardiogenic shock, and most of them die as its consequence.

Cardiogenic shock occurs when the heart can no longer maintain its pumping action because of heart muscle damage. Blood pressure falls, fatally starving vital areas like the kidneys and the brain. Once the heart muscle damage spreads, and the heart is not able to pump properly, all body systems quickly deteriorate and the person dies.

In the operation pioneered by Dr. Adrian Kantrowitz of Sinai Hospital of Detroit, a mechanical assistance is provided to the weakened heart muscle, allowing it to recover its normal strength.

The procedure is simple and can be performed at the patient's bedside. A long, narrow, plastic balloon is inserted into the artery in the leg through a small incision done under local anesthesia. The balloon is passed up the artery and

---

Additional material touching on this subject can be found in chapters 7, 24, 32, 84, 94, 96 and 99.

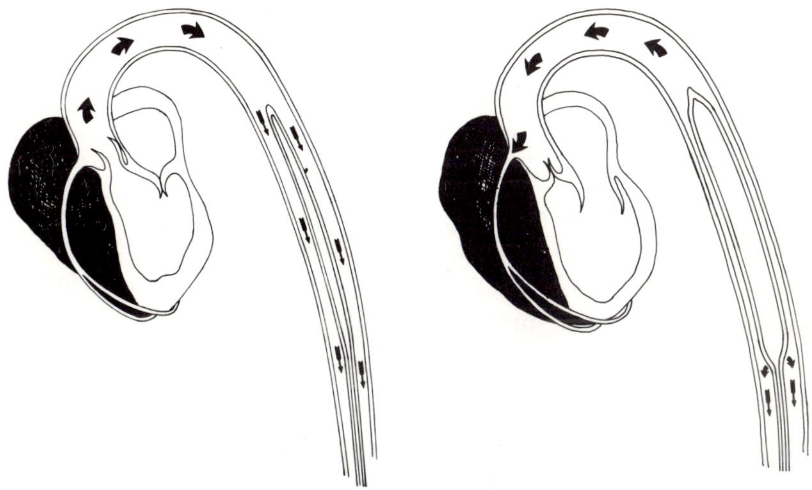

A balloon pump in position in the descending thoracic aorta. To the left, the balloon is seen in deflated position, permitting normal outflow of the blood from the ventricle. To the right, the balloon is inflated as the heart relaxes and the ventricles fill with blood.

brought into position in the upper part of the aorta, the main artery of the body.

The balloon is attached to a catheter (tube) which ends in a valve that remains outside the body. Once the balloon is in position, the valve is attached to a machine called the Kantrowitz Drive Unit, which inflates or deflates the balloon in rhythm with the heart beat.

The action of the balloon is electronically synchronized with the action of the heart, and each time the balloon inflates, it gives an extra boost to the circulation, allowing the heart to recover its normal strength slowly. Once the continuously-run tests show that the heart is again functioning normally, the pumping is stopped and the balloon withdrawn.

Cardiogenic shock can occur soon after the heart attack or it can happen after a lapse of many hours. If the shock occurs within 30 hours after the heart attack, it is called an early shock; if it happens more than 30 hours after the attack, it is called a delayed shock. The balloon pumping is not effective for the treatment of delayed shock, but in the cases of early shock the results have been very good.

Reporting on the results of his technique to a group of 25 patients suffering from early shock, Dr. Kantrowitz notes that 90% of the patients came out of the shock during balloon pumping. Eleven of them, 45%, recovered from their heart attacks and were discharged from the hospital.

88. REMOVING KIDNEYS FOR REPAIRS

TWO OPERATIONS in which a diseased kidney was removed from the patient, its defects corrected, and then returned as a healthy organ to the body, were recently performed by Dr. Russell K. Lawson of the University of Oregon Medical School in Portland. This is the first time that such operations have been performed.

The new technique allows the surgeon to perform delicate repairs on the artery in the kidney which would be impossible to do if the kidney could not be removed from the body. Under these conditions, the surgeon is not rushed, and he can use very fine sutures, and small instruments which would be impossible to use inside the body.

After the kidneys are removed, they are flushed out and cooled. The surgeon then does the required repair work leisurely since the kidneys can be preserved outside the body for six to eight hours without damage. This is very important because the work to be done by the surgeon must be meticulous, and it requires quite a bit of time. After the repair work on the kidney is completed, the organ is returned to the body and sewed in. Unlike with transplants, there is no danger of rejection since a person's own kidney is being put back into his body.

In the first operation which Dr. Lawson performed, he removed the kidneys from a 31-year-old man who had blood

Additional material touching on this subject can be found in chapters 52 and 54.

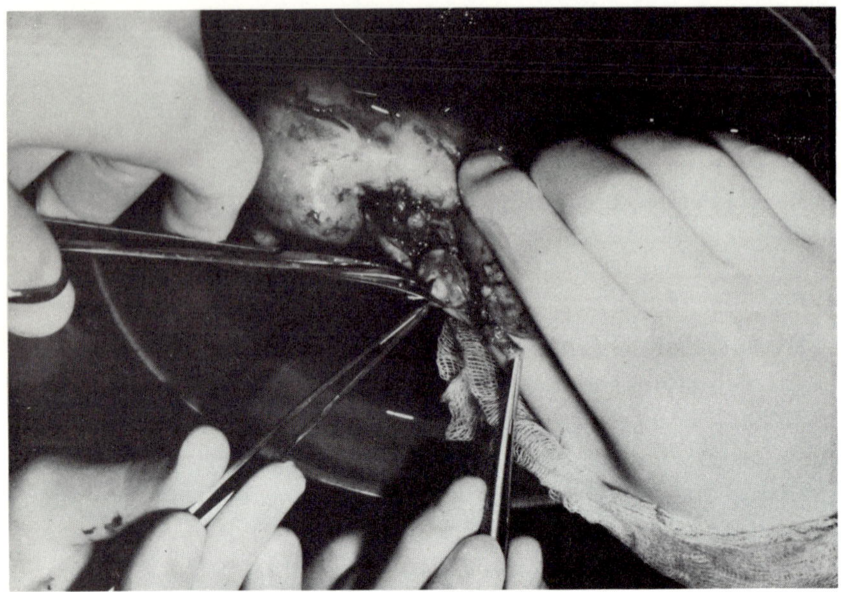

The aneurism of a kidney being opened during an operation.

in the urine resulting from an *aneurysm* (a blood-containing tumor) in the kidney artery. In this case, the diseased portion was cut away, and the artery repaired.

The second case involved a 21-year-old woman with a five-year history of severe high blood pressure. Examination showed that the artery in her right kidney was completely blocked. Her high blood pressure was being caused by the condition of her kidney. The blocked artery was cleaned out and her blood pressure returned to normal.

Dr. Lawson's new technique of kidney removal opens up the possibility of using it to examine the kidney in suspected cases of cancer of the kidney. In such cases, the kidney could be removed from the patient, carefully examined, and then replaced if a tumor is not found and cancer is ruled out.

89. A "SAFESLEEPER" BABY MATTRESS

A CLEVERLY-DESIGNED, two-part baby mattress is now being sold in England, designed especially for babies who lie on their stomachs.

The new mattress is skillfully designed to allow babies to breathe freely and without risk when sleeping face down. The main feature of the mattress is that it comes in two sections. The detachable top part—the self-ventilating "pillow" section—is made of aerated ridge foam rubber, with a slip-on cellular, cotton cover which provides both additional air circulation and continuity with the main section of the mattress.

The two-section mattress also makes cleaning easier for mothers, allowing easy removal of the portion of mattress—the head—which requires the most frequent attention. The head section is held in place with fasteners, is easily detachable and is fully washable, insuring maximum bed hygiene. The main section of the mattress is covered with a pretty rose-patterned easily washed polyvinyl. It is not quite so thick as an ordinary baby mattress, but that means it is less bulky and easier to handle. Babies seem quite comfortable on it.

The Safesleeper mattress is available in both baby bed and pram sizes. Some doctors—and parents—feel that a tiny baby shouldn't be put in a large baby bed during the early weeks,

Additional material touching on this subject can be found in chapter 22.

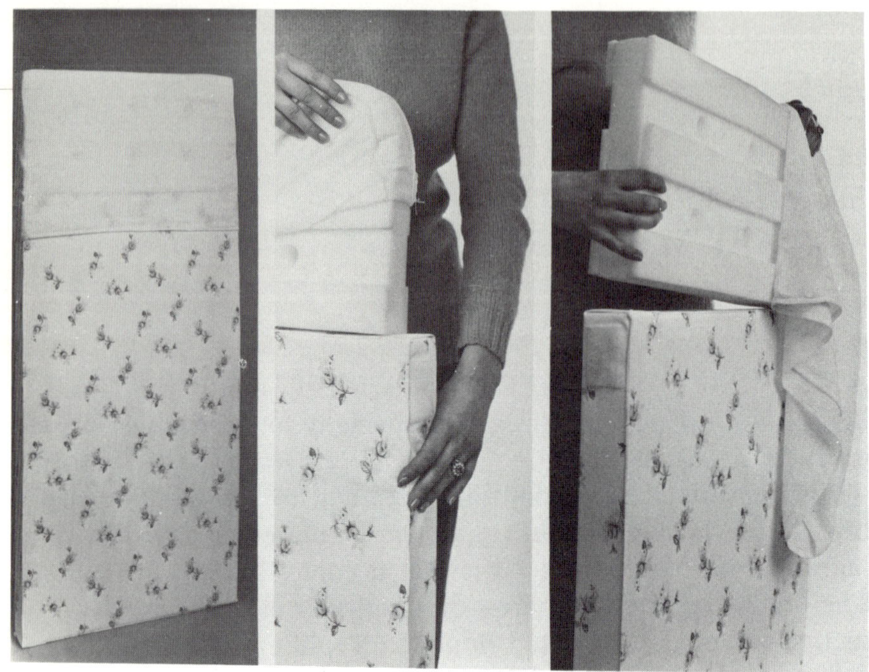

The standard size Safesleeper mattress. The pads on the sides of the main section grip the cover of the pillow section and hold it tightly in place.

because it feels more secure in a smaller crib. Pillows are "out" at this early stage, but if a mother using a regular baby bed is anxious over the fact that the baby is sleeping face down, the use of the new British mattress could relieve her of many worries.

The Safesleeper mattress is made by Price Bros. & Co., Ltd., Wellington, Somerset, England. In England, the regular-size mattress sells for about $13, the pram unit for about $6.

90. REPLANTING PARTS OF THE HUMAN BODY

REPLANTING PARTS of the human body means taking a part of the body that has been cut off and putting it back where it belongs.

It's easy to have a part of the body cut away. By accident you can cut your finger off. Your leg could get crushed in an accident and the doctors might have to cut it off. Your hand could get caught in a machine in the factory and be severed.

Commonly, people who have lost parts of their bodies have them replaced by artificial parts, called prostheses. An artificial arm or leg is not the best solution, and that is why surgeons have been trying to figure out a way to replant the actual arm or leg or limb that people lose in accidents.

Of course, is it not sufficient to simply take a hand that was cut off and stitch it back to the arm. The organ that was cut off is dead. There is no life in it. There is no blood in it. It has no feeling. When the hand is replanted, it must also be regenerated—it must be brought back to life.

This is very difficult. When an arm is cut off, everything in it is disconnected from the rest of the body. The bone is cut, the nerves are cut, the veins are cut. To replant the arm, the ends of the cut bones have to be put together correctly and all the nerves and veins have to be sewn together accurately.

Additional material touching on this subject can be found in chapters 63 and 80.

There are two big problems in replanting parts of the body. One problem is that the body often rejects the severed part after it has been stitched back on. The body refuses to let it come to life again. Another problem is that the severed part must be kept fresh while it is disconnected or it cannot be replanted.

These two problems were so difficult to solve that doctors all over the world were not able to solve them for hundreds of years.

But about ten years ago, in 1962, two doctors in Boston, Massachusetts, Dr. Ronald A. Malt and Dr. William H. Harris, finally managed to replant a human arm. It was a great step forward in surgery.

The first person to have a replanted arm was a 12-year-old boy. The boy, Everett Knowles, Jr., fell under a train, and the wheels of the train sliced off his right arm, just below the shoulder. Everett's arm was stitched back on by the two doctors and it grew back perfectly. Today, Everett can use it on his job like any other young man. He can even lift a pail full of water with it.

What was the secret that these two doctors discovered? Why couldn't doctors replant arms before? Dr. Malt and Dr. Harris discovered that to replant the arm they had to perform the operation in reverse. Previously, doctors stitched the veins together as soon as they replanted a part of a body because they wanted the blood to flow through it again as soon as possible. But this turned out to be the wrong first step. The first step was to join the cut bones.

Since Everett's arm was replanted, about 809 cases of limb rejoining have been reported throughout the entire world. There has been about 65% success in rejoining but function has often been less than desirable because limbs torn off are usually severely damaged. In the last two or three years microsurgery techniques have been used in the replant operations. Medical authorities expect results to improve using microsurgery.

Doctors are very hopeful that since we have learned how to "replant" arms and hands successfully, in the future it will be possible to "transplant" arms and hands just as now we transplant kidneys or corneas. If that becomes possible, many people will get back their lost limbs.

Today, it is only possible to replant a limb that has not been damaged too badly. An arm that has been crushed cannot be replanted. In the future it may be possible to transplant such an arm from a dead person so that a living person may continue to enjoy his life to the fullest.

91. ELECTROSLEEP

FOR THE PAST 20 years, a type of electrical treatment called electrosleep has been used in Russia. This is a method of inducing a relaxed state of sleep by the use of a very low intensity electric current sent through the head. In recent years, the treatment has also been used in Austria and West Germany, and now, it is being used in America.

Under a patent licensing deal with the Russians, a transistorized, battery-operated, portable Electrosom "sleep machine," that is now being widely used in Russia, has been sold to more than 125 practicing physicians in this country.

Doctors are reporting they are finding electrosleep to be particularly well suited for the treatment of all the diseases having an anxiety or psychogenic origin or overlay. This is much in line with the claims advanced for the machine.

According to Dr. Paul Williamson, of Euless, Texas, the machine is just a square wave generator made up of the best available materials. "These square waves are very similar to sleep waves generated in mid-brain," explains Dr. Williamson. "We are certain electrosleep creates natural sleep waves in the brain. Why the brain is a copycat about sleep waves, we do not know. When real sleep waves are put into the mid-brain, the patient very definitely gets drowsy. In just a few minutes the patient's own body begins making sleep waves. The body's own sleep waves continue for quite a while. This is

---

Additional material touching on this subject can be found in chapters 48, 57, 67 and 85.

one reason electrosleep is so useful. A short application will last from three to ten hours."

The dose can vary from slight tranquilization to deep sleep. In general, tranquilization can be obtained in a 5-10 minute application and gentle sleep in 20-30 minutes. Deep sleep is rarely used. There is no chance of an overdose—a patient can be awakened by simply shaking him gently by the shoulder. The equipment can be operated by any intelligent person. The electrodes, placed over the eyes and the back of the head, cause no discomfort and are not dangerous to the eyes.

The interesting thing about the treatment is that the patient can get up from a treatment, go about his business for an hour or two, and then go home—and to sleep! "It seems," says Dr. Williamson, "a love affair springs up immediately" the moment the patient sees the bed.

Electrosleep in about 30-minute doses is reported to relieve insomniacs. After an evening treatment, the patient goes home and goes to sleep. "You can change people's habits of sleeping with two or three weeks of electrosleep treatments," asserts Dr. Williamson. "At least 70% will get in the habit of retiring and falling into a sound, sound sleep."

Good results are reported in treatment of tension headaches and menstrual cramps. A tranquilizing dose of 10-20 minutes will relieve the psychic overlay in menstrual cramps. The tension headache is affected in the same way. The versatility of the treatment is illustrated in the fact that good results have been reported in the treatment of psychogenic asthma, where one can achieve easy breathing in 3-5 minutes.

Neither the doctors using the machines now nor clinical researchers have reported any toxic effects or contraindications. The machine can be used in almost any place as one would use a tranquilizer or a sedative. There is no "drunken sedation" effect and the treatment is non-addictive, because addiction to sleep waves is normal.

92. NEW RELIEF FOR SEVERE ARTHRITIS

A GROUP OF BRITISH DOCTORS at Stoke Mandeville Hospital in Aylesbury, which specializes in the treatment of arthritis and rheumatism, have announced some very encouraging results in tests of a new treatment for severe, crippling arthritis.

The drug itself isn't new, but its use against arthritis on a huge scale is. The drug is *penicillamine*, a chemical compound which can be derived from either natural or synthetic penicillin but which doesn't act as an antibiotic itself. For some years penicillamine has been used for treating lead poisoning, and also in the treatment of a rare illness known as Wilson's Disease in which large amounts of copper accumulate in the body, and create a dangerous situation.

Penicillamine is effective in these conditions because it soaks up lead, copper and other metals, and converts them to new harmless compounds. But despite the fact that it was already a familiar drug to doctors, they still do not know how or why it relieves the symptoms of arthritis.

Penicillamine was first tested against arthritis because doctors thought it might be effective in breaking up molecules of a complex (protein) compound called *rheumatoid factor*, which is always formed in rheumatic joints, and which may be the cause of some of the pain suffered by arthritics. Because it provided striking relief in some very severe cases, British doctors in five hospitals in different cities decided to organize a proper test of the drug under the direction of the Stoke Mandeville Hospital.

The results of the trial showed that the patients treated with penicillamine had improved. They had less pain and swelling in their joints, took less time to loosen up in the morning, had stronger grips, were able to perform certain tasks more easily, were less anaemic, and showed improvement in laboratory tests.

These results were particularly striking because (as is usual with a new drug) the patients undergoing the new treatment were all extreme cases for whom all other available forms of treatment had proven virtually useless. Doctors now plan to extend the use of penicillamine to larger numbers of patients with less severe arthritis.

The drug may be effective for several reasons. It may attack micro-organisms causing arthritis—if, as some suspect, this is the cause of arthritis. Or, it may be effective because it suppresses the human body's immune reaction—its protective reaction against foreign organisms. It may be preventing what is called an *auto-immune* reaction by which the human body mistakenly damages its own tissues. The idea that arthritis is an auto-immune disease is becoming increasingly popular.

Penicillamine has one big disadvantage. About 30% of arthritis patients have to be taken off it because of two occasional harmful side-effects: damage to the kidneys and damage to the tiny blood cells called *platelets*. However, while these side effects may restrict its use, doctors are confident from the tests to date that the side effects can be detected early enough to avoid permanent damage to the patient.

93. AUSTRALIAN PILL
BATTLES BREAST CANCER

AN AUSTRALIAN medical research team is developing a pill which could revolutionize the treatment of breast cancer in women.

The work is being done at the Garvan Institute of Medical Research in Sydney by a three-man team led by the institute's director, Dr. Leslie Lazarus. The team has begun testing the breast cancer pill on humans, following an extensive and successful series of tests on rats.

Success of the project would dramatically affect the lives of many thousands of women around the world. In Australia alone, it is estimated that one out of every 18 women will contract breast cancer during her lifetime.

The pill would replace major surgery, an operation which involves removal of the pituitary gland from the base of the brain, and which is so serious that it is usually performed only as a last resort—when the cancer has spread to other parts of the body.

The purpose of the operation is to rid the body of hormones released by the pituitary. Although the various hormones produced by the pituitary are important in body development, one of them, *prolactin*, is known to be involved in the growth of breast cancer and another, the human growth hormone, is also suspect.

Instead of undergoing major surgery to remove these two

hormones, the patient would be able to suppress them by taking the pill.

Dr. Lazarus and his team have already produced a number of synthetic compounds which block the release of prolactin and growth hormone.

"The idea is to use the compounds in pill form to stop the secretion of prolactin and the growth hormone," Dr. Lazarus explains. "Some of our compounds act only on prolactin, some act only on the growth hormone, while others act on both.

"They have worked very successfully in blocking the secretion of prolactin and the growth hormone in rats without any deleterious side-effects.

"We have now started tests on human volunteers to see if they produce the same results. These tests will be extended until we find the most effective compound."

Dr. Lazarus said it would be at least another five years before his team could be completely sure that the pill's long-term effects are beneficial.

"Decreasing the hormone level in the patient is only the first step," he said. "We must be able to maintain this effect."

Dr. Lazarus points out that one of the big problems with the pituitary operation is that only about half the patients who underwent surgery responded to it. There was no way, at the moment, of predicting who would, and who would not, respond.

He said that the new compounds could be used in the short term to see if a patient was likely to respond to surgery. If her condition improved with suppression of the hormones, she would then be a good candidate for an operation.

Dr. Lazarus hopes that the pill will eventually completely eliminate the need for surgery.

94. A "PACEMAKER"
FOR DISABLED BRAINS

A "BRAIN PACEMAKER" that helps in certain types of involuntary movement disorders has been developed by Dr. Irving S. Cooper, Director of Neurological Surgery at the St. Barnabas Hospital, Bronx, New York. Some 20 years ago, Dr. Cooper was the first to use surgery in the treatment of Parkinson's disease, and recently he has developed a new technique of brain freeze in the treatment of stroke victims (which is described in Chapter 74).

So far, Dr. Cooper has used the pacemaker to treat intractable epilepsy and spastic conditions of various origins. Reporting on 12 spastic patients, Dr. Cooper reported significant improvement in seven out of 10 patients, and moderate improvement in two others.

One 50-year-old man who was unable to bend his right elbow and knee since the age of three can now bend both the knee and the elbow and walk for the first time without a cane. A 12-year-old boy with cerebral palsy, who was unable to sit up alone and was totally incapacitated by bilateral spacticity (paralyses on both sides of the body), can now sit up alone, propel his wheelchair unaided, and partially feed himself.

The new procedure involves implanting in the brain a silicon-coated mesh plate with four or eight pairs of platinum

Additional material touching on this subject can be found in chapters 7, 24, 32, 84, 96, 98 and 99.

disc electrodes. An antenna is implanted under the skin of the chest, and the electrodes are activated by a current charge sent through the skin. A battery-powered transmitter, small enough to be carried in the patient's pocket, turns the implanted pacer on and off. The duration of individual electric stimulation varies from ten minutes each hour during waking hours, to ten-minute intervals, on and off around the clock.

The patients included in this study have been treated for varying periods of time, up to one year. "Improvement is progressive, at least for the first three months of stimulation," reported Dr. Cooper. There have been no adverse reactions on the physical, intellectual or behavioral function of the patients.

The new study is only the "seed" stage of the investigation of this new method of brain stimulation. Dr. Cooper hopes that further studies will bring even better results.

95. A HELP FOR STUBBORN EPILEPSY IN CHILDREN

IMIPRAMINE HYDROCHLORIDE (Tofranil), a drug originally used for mental depression treatment, may help at least some sufferers from otherwise unyielding seizures.

Dr. Gerhard H. Fromm, and other doctors at the University of Pittsburgh School of Medicine, report using imipramine in 20 children with *petit mal* and minor motor seizures who failed to benefit from conventional anti-convulsant drugs, or had become resistant to them. Fifteen of the children, who ranged in age from three months to 14 years, responded well to the new drug.

Imipramine was given to the children by mouth, with doses increased gradually. The young patients were carefully observed by their parents and teachers.

The initial response to the treatment with the anti-depressant was so good that 11 children had a 90% or better reduction in seizures, but in some patients the improvement was only temporary. Nine of the 15 children had recurrences of their minor motor or *petit mal* seizures. However, the other six have continued to show significant improvement for three years so far.

Six children whose seizures have decreased also became brighter, according to their parents, and appeared more alert

---

Additional material touching on this subject can be found in chapters 94 and 98.

during follow-up examinations. Those who were attending school or special-education classes showed considerable improvement in their school work. One 12-year-old was able to benefit from instruction for the first time in his life.

Further studies are now being carried out with this drug on epilepsy patients, but the results of the treatment of the first 20 patients suggest that imipramine has good value in the treatment of *petit mal* or minor motor seizures. Since this drug has also been used for the past 10 years in the treatment of children with enuresis (incontinence) it appears to be safe in children as well as in adult patients.

96. ATOMIC PACEMAKERS: SAFE WAY TO A LONGER LIFE

HEART PACEMAKERS powered with atomic power are here to stay—they have passed their tests. Soon, they will be widely available to anyone who needs a heart pacemaker.

The atomic powered pacemaker is different from an ordinary pacemaker only in that it runs longer before it has to be replaced with a new one—but that is a very important difference.

A conventional heart pacemaker has to be replaced every two years, while the atomic model runs ten years. This means one replacement operation every ten years, instead of five over the same period of time.

Because of the reduced number of required replacement operations, the atomic pacemaker increases a patient's chances of survival five times, according to Dr. Paul Laurens, the French cardiologist who developed the first atomic pacemaker.

The nuclear pacemaker is powered with a pinch of Plutonium-238, a deadly, radioactive material, safely enclosed in a special capsule which has been extensively tested for safety. Great care has been taken to ensure that not a bit of the deadly radioactive poison will escape from it. The capsules have been tested by crushing them with ten-thousand-pound loads, shooting at them with revolvers, shooting them into

Additional material touching on this subject can be found in chapters 7, 24, 32, 84, 94, 98 and 99.

steel plates at 120 m.p.h., and burning them in fires reaching the temperature of 2,400° F. These were just some of the stringent tests that were required by the Atomic Energy Commission before they permitted the atomic powered pacemakers to be used in this country.

The radioactive material is so well "packaged" that it is completely safe for the wearer. At the surface of the pacemaker, the maximum amount of radiation is about the same as that emitted by a wristwatch with a luminous (radium) dial. Over the period of a year, the radiation at the skin was measured as about the same as that generated in a single diagnostic X-ray.

The atomic powered pacemakers were first used in France, in 1970, and a number of them were implanted in various European countries—particularly in West Germany—before the first U.S. atomic pacemaker was implanted in a patient, in July, 1972, at the Buffalo, N.Y., Veterans Administration Hospital.

Since the atomic pacemaker was first implanted, a total of 150 volunteers in different countries have been equipped with the new device, and to date there have been no problems of failure of the pacemaker in a wearer.

Though the average age of the wearers is near 40, they have been implanted in young persons as well. Dr. Laurens has implanted plutonium-powered pacemakers in two girls, aged 10 and 11, and a nine-year-old boy has had an atomic pacemaker implanted in Czechoslovakia. For a young person, with a life expectancy of 70, the new device makes an enormous difference: It means having to submit to five or six replacement operations instead of 30.

The cost of the nuclear pacer is about three times as much as the conventional model, but wearers will save money because of the reduced number of required replacement operations.

97. ELECTRONIC STIMULATOR FOR PARALYZED FOOT

ONE AFTER-EFFECT of a stroke can be a paralyzed foot. Medically, the condition is called a *spastic equinovarus foot*, meaning a club foot caused by a stroke.

The afflicted person has a twisted foot—pointed either to the left or right. He drags the foot because he has lost *volitional control* over the leg —control exercised by the brain.

The severity of the condition varies. If the degree of the paralysis is severe, besides being twisted down and in, the foot may also tip sideways. In such cases the weight must be borne on the edge of the foot. Also, the toes may claw, making walking painful as well as difficult.

The most common treatment for this condition is a short leg brace, but if the paralysis is severe, the foot continues to twist inside the brace and surgery is often necessary. Various surgical procedures: tendon lengthening, heel cord lengthening, tendon transfers, and combinations of these procedures are used to correct the deformity.

However, many stroke victims are older persons with circulation problems, blood vessel diseases, and diabetes—conditions that might make this type of surgery impossible. Also, because of the difficulty in getting proper balance of action in the leg muscles, the results of surgical procedures are

---

Additional material touching on this subject can be found in chapter 31.

usually unpredictable, and repeated operations may be required to obtain good results.

Now, a team of physicians at Rancho Los Amigos Hospital at Downey, California, led by Dr. Robert Waters, orthopedic surgeon, and Dr. Donald McNeal, an engineer, developed an implantable electronic stimulator which stimulates the nerves in the paralyzed foot bringing the foot into the normal position during walking.

The stimulator works by stimulating the *peroneal nerve*—the outer nerve in the lower leg. The system consists of a stimulator, an antenna, a flexible lead, a receiver, an electrode and a heel switch.

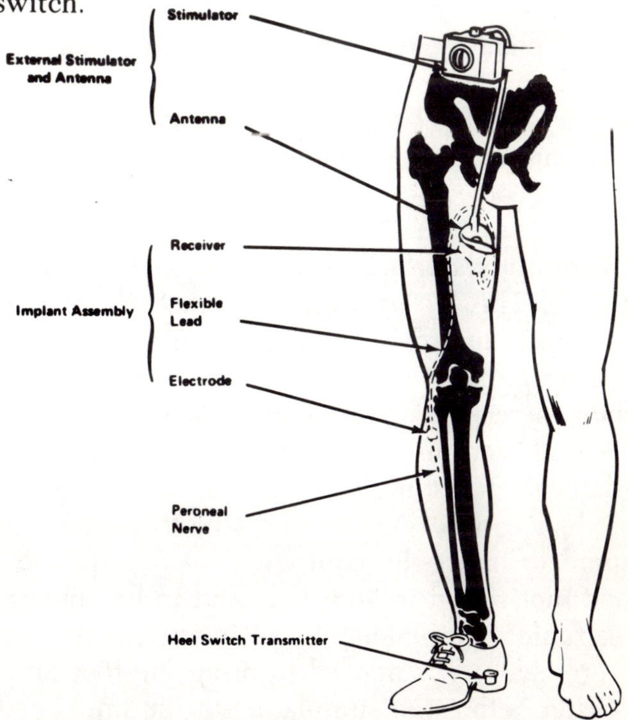

The external stimulator is suspended on a belt on the waist in a position that the patient can conveniently reach. The external antenna is worn under the clothes and attached to the leg over the implanted receiver with tape or adhesive spray.

A tiny radio receiver is implanted under the skin, inside the upper part of the thigh. Another cut is made in the outside of the lower leg, and the electrode is implanted encircling the peroneal nerve. The receiver and the electrode are connected with the lead, placed under the skin. A round disc antenna is taped to the skin over the receiver (with tape or spray adhesive), and connected to the stimulator, which is worn on the patient's belt. The heel switch, which is a small switch and transmitting device, is mounted in the heel of the patient's shoe.

When the patient lifts his heel, the heel switch signals the stimulator to send a radio frequency signal through the skin to the implanted receiver, which, through the electrode, stimulates the nerve with a "shock." This causes the appropriate muscles to contract, bringing the foot up and outward into its approximately normal walking position. When the heel comes down again, the stimulation is stopped until the patient again lifts the heel to take another step.

The stimulator also has a unique feature—an exercising module. This automatically contracts the muscles at regular intervals to improve muscle tone, strength and appearance. It requires no action by the patient—he can read or watch TV while exercise takes place automatically.

Not all persons with a stroke-paralyzed foot are good candidates for the stimulator. In order to be able to benefit from the device, a person must be able to tolerate the surgery required to insert the equipment in the leg and must have a good motivation to adjust to, and to be able to operate, the electronic equipment. Sometimes, when the paralysis is severe, surgery is needed to bring the foot into a functional position before the stimulator can be implanted.

Over the past three years, some 35 patients have been fitted with these stimulators at the Downey Hospital.

98. NEW TECHNIQUES HELP CONTROL EPILEPSY

TREATMENT OF EPILEPSY has followed a conventional procedure for so many years that some doctors are not even aware that new treatment techniques have been developed in recent years.

Two important, new techniques are *gas liquid chromatography* (GLC), also known as *serum scan*, and *telemetry*.

The GLC procedure is a study of the person's serum samples (fluid samples from the spinal column) performed with special equipment. It is in operation in only about a dozen institutions in the U.S. and in only one in Canada. These neurological treatment and research centers will do studies for out-of-town doctors who mail in fluid samples.

The GLC equipment measures drug levels in the patient's serum. Through this procedure the doctor can learn immediately which anticonvulsant drug is best for his patient and the most effective dosage to prescribe. Anticonvulsant drugs are a problem because they have to be prescribed in increasing doses until seizures are under control, or until they become toxic (poisonous) to the patient. GLC eliminates these problems.

Telemetry involves the use of closed-circuit TV and split-screen units on which both the patient and his EEG (brain wave test) results can be seen by the doctor at the same time.

Additional material touching on this subject can be found in chapters 94 and 95.

According to Dr. Gilbert H. Glaser, Professor and Chairman of the Department of Neurology at Yale University, the use of telemetry to observe patients outside the laboratory conditions is proving very valuable. Merely having the patient to be observed placed in a hospital ward with other patients, has led to discovery of changes in his EEG. "Social situations exist in the ward," notes Dr. Glaser, "which do not happen in the laboratory, and these cause stresses which can be observed in the EEG."

Like GLC, telemetry is usually available only in the special neurologic centers, but doctors in other areas can send their patients to these centers for observation and receive a plan of treatment worked out on the basis of GLC and telemetry studies.

99. MIDGET ELECTROCARDIOGRAPH BENEFITS HEART PATIENTS

THE DEVELOPMENT of a portable midget electrocardiograph has long been sought so that a heart patient could carry the device on his person and promptly record the condition of his heart in case of cardiac disturbance, facilitating the doctor's diagnosis and treatment.

Efforts to reduce the size of an electrocardiograph have made considerable progress, and it is well known that small devices of this kind are used to check the electrocardiograms of astronauts. Moreover, small portable electrocardiographs for cardiac patients are also in use. But all of these devices, though reduced in size, are still too bulky and heavy to be carried around easily.

Moreover, cardiac fits, such as angina pectoris and arrhythmia, occur suddenly but disappear in a short time, leaving the heart in normal condition. Therefore, under the conventional system whereby the heart patient must go to his hospital for an electrocardiograph test, the condition of his heart at the time of a seizure cannot be recorded. This has been a major obstacle to the diagnosis and treatment of heart trouble.

If the purpose is to obtain an electrocardiogram only for the duration of a cardiac fit, the heart condition need not necessarily be recorded for a long time. In most cases, only 30

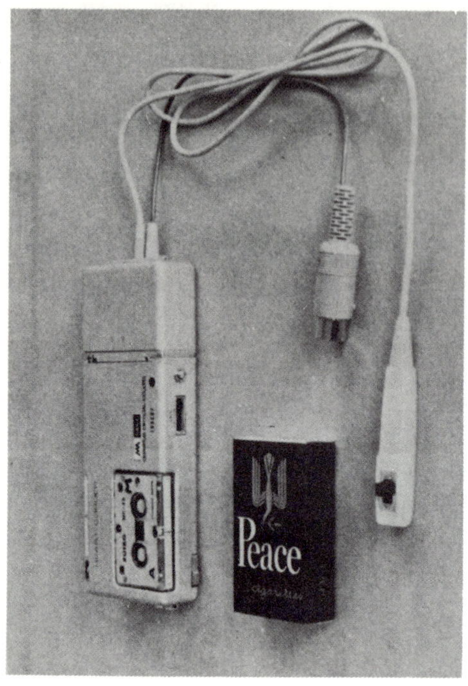

The newly developed midget electrocardiograph is slightly larger than a pack of cigarettes.

seconds to several minutes of recording is enough for diagnosis.

Recently, a device of super-mini size was developed in Japan by a group led by Prof. Eiichi Kimura of the Nippon Medical School.

The newly developed midget electrocardiograph enables the bearer to turn it on to record his heart condition anywhere, as soon as he is stricken.

The device, an improvement of the cassette tape recorder, is only six inches long, 2.3 inches wide, 0.87 inches thick, and weighs a mere 8.8 ounces. It can be carried in a pocket or a handbag. In the event of a cardiac seizure, all the patient has to do is to attach the electrodes at the end of cords leading out of the device to the right and left chest with adhesive tape and turn it on.

The heartbeat, expressed as the intensity of electric current, is recorded on a tape, which is taken to a hospital. The recorded pulsation is reproduced with a demodulator and observed with the aid of a cathode ray tube or transferred onto ordinary electrocardiogram paper.

The new electrocardiograph is suitable for those patients who complain of severe palpitations, arrhythmia, chest pains and a sense of oppression or discomfort in the chest and whose fits cannot be conclusively diagnosed by an electrocardiogram recorded during their normal condition.

Professor Kimura's group has reported that the new devices, now being carried since the summer of 1972 by 55 outpatients of a hospital attached to the Nippon Medical School, have all produced accurate electrocardiograms, making it possible to pinpoint defective areas in the hearts of 34 patients suffering from angina pectoris or arrhythmia.

100. NEW LANGUAGE
FOR HANDICAPPED CHILDREN

RONNIE, A SPASTIC DEAF-MUTE boy at a day center in Melbourne, and Andrew, a silent six-year-old pupil at the Windgap Subnormal School, Sydney, are just two of a growing number of handicapped Australian children discovering the excitement of communication.

Denied normal speech, they are learning how to "speak" through the use of a system of symbols, a universal pictorial language invented by Mr. Charles K. Bliss, a retired chemical engineer from Vienna who now lives in Sydney.

Semantography—one writing for one world—or *Blissymbolics*, as he now prefers to call it, was intended by him to become the means of free communication between the diverse races of the planet; and indeed Charles Bliss still hopes that it will become so.

"But now it has been found how immediately useful my picture-writing is as an aid to communication for handicapped children," he said. "This is already a reward beyond my expectations."

Now being used by crippled and paralyzed children at the Ontario Crippled Children's Centre, Toronto, Canada as well as in parts of Australia, semantography is essentially a system of simple, pictorial symbols of writing, typing, and printing

---

Additional material touching on this subject can be found in chapter 83.

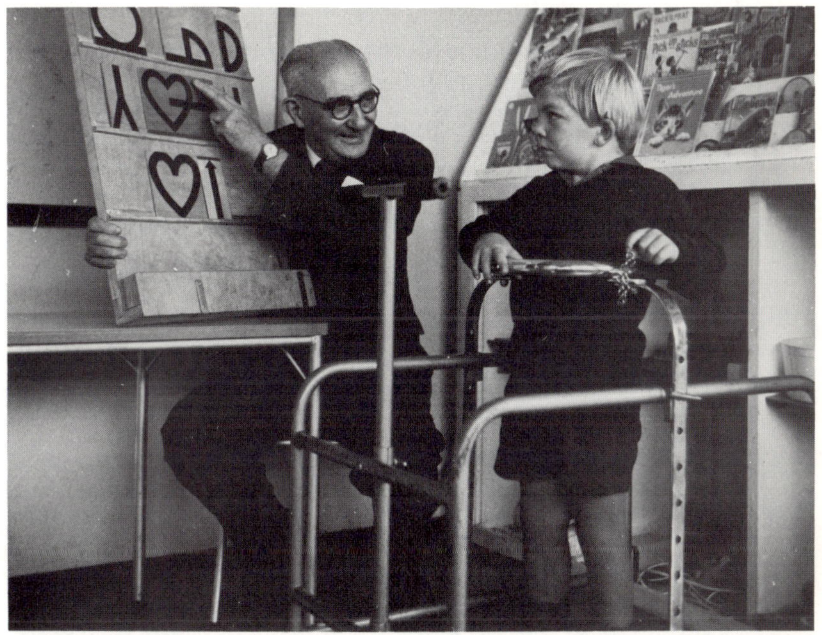

Pictorial symbols for ground, sun, morning, day, evening, moon, and "man loves woman" are a first step in helping a six year-old emerge from a wall of silence.

that can be read by speakers of any language, without any need of translation.

The system also contains, according to its inventor, simple semantics and symbolic language which even children can learn to apply to their problems. Moreover, when normal utterances are "translated" into Blissymbolics, their basic truths—or lack of them—stand clearly revealed.

In Charles Bliss' pictorial alphabet, there are some 100 basic symbols, 30 of which (Arabic numerals, mathematical signs, punctuation, directional indicators and so on) are already recognized internationally.

"Man" is represented by an inverted "Y." "Ground" or "earth" has for its symbol a short, horizontal line; a dot placed above this indicates "above," "upper," and so on; if the dot is placed under the line, the meanings include "below," "lower," etc.

Other Blissymbolics include a circle for "sun," or "day;" a small circle for "mouth;" and a small circle with a dot in it for "eye." Many of the pictographs blend to yield new concepts —"mouth" and "ear" combined gives the symbol readily recognized as "language." Then, this new symbol in conjunction with the zig-zag "lightning" ("electricity") symbol yields "telephone;" and the picture writing for "television" is, quite logically, "eye" plus a box shape, plus "ear," plus "electricity."

Even such abstract concepts as "tolerance" can be easily conveyed in picture form. The Blissymbol for "reason" (as well as for "skull") is a horizontal open half-circle. Inside this is drawn a plus-minus sign, and an exclamation mark is put after the whole. The plus-minus sign, of course, already indicates the notion of "tolerance" to mathematicians and engineers.

Charles Bliss is excited about the possibilities of his "alphabet" being used by handicapped children. For children in wheel chairs there is a semi-circular table top of wood and glass on which 15 or more basic symbols can be arrayed. Paralyzed children soon learn how to move a radial pointer to indicate their messages to a world that, until now, could not hear their voices.

For Ronnie and Andrew and hundreds of other children like them, the picture language of Charles Bliss provides a new gift of human contact.

INDEX

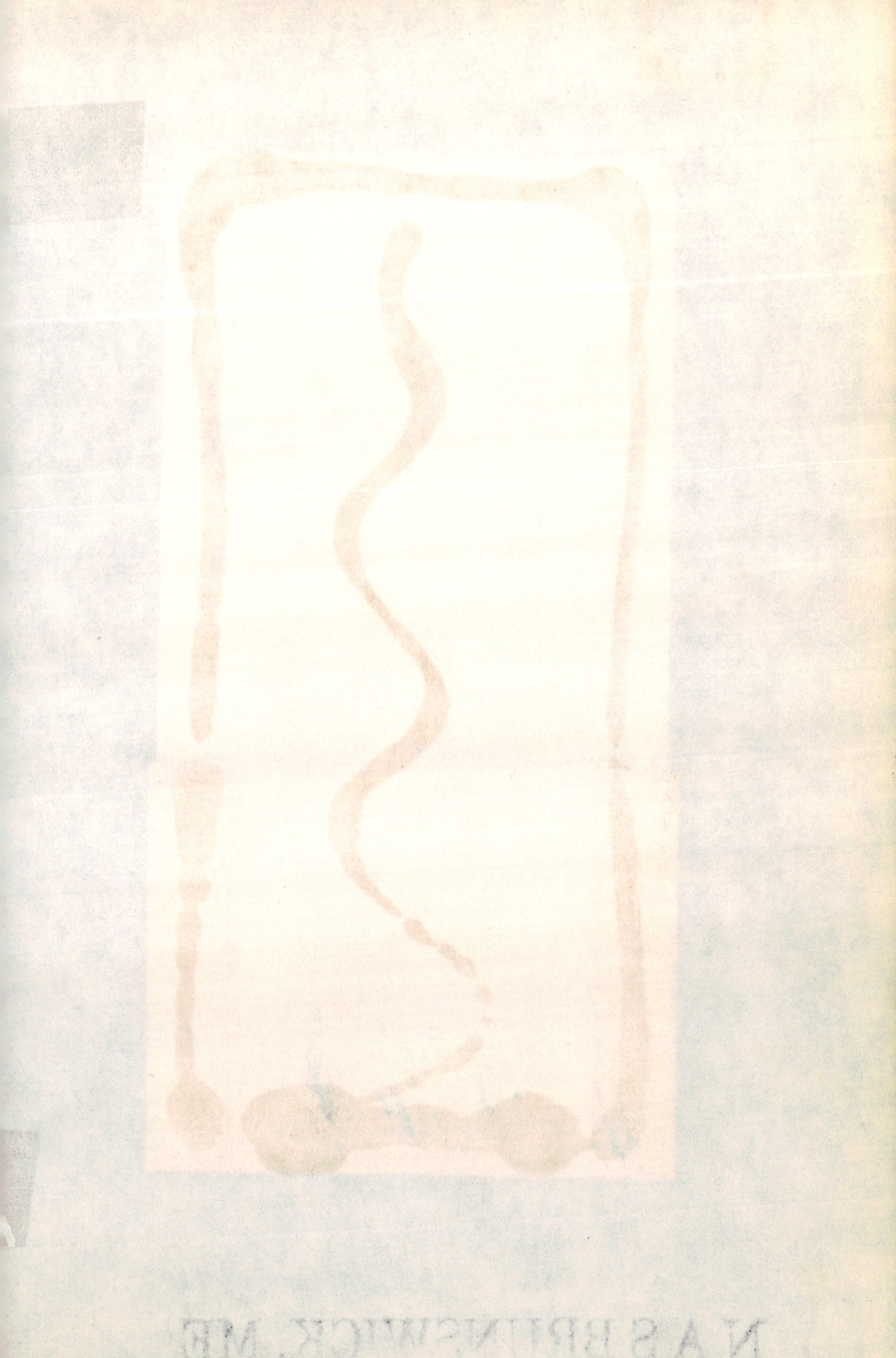